The Second Sin

Thomas Szasz is Professor of Psychiatry at the State University of New York Upstate Medical Center in Syracuse, New York. He is a member of the editorial board of *The Humanist, Journal of Humanistic Psychology, Journal of Drug Addiction,* and *Contemporary Psychoanalysis,* and of the board of consultants of *The Psychoanalytic Review;* a member of the American Psychoanalytic Association; a fellow of the American Psychiatric Association and the Royal Society of Health (London); a consultant to the Committee on Mental Hygiene of the New York State Bar Association; and a co-founder and Chairman of the Board of Directors of the American Association for the Abolition of Involuntary Mental Hospitalization. He is the author of more than two hundred articles and book reviews, and of nine books, including *The Myth of Mental Illness, Ideology and Insanity, The Manufacture of Madness,* and *The Age of Madness.*

The Second Sin

THOMAS SZASZ

ANCHOR BOOKS
ANCHOR PRESS / DOUBLEDAY
GARDEN CITY, NEW YORK
1974

THE SECOND SIN
was originally published in a hardcover edition by
Anchor Press/Doubleday & Company, Inc. in 1973.

Anchor Books Edition: 1974

ISBN: 0-385-04638-3

TO MY MOTHER

Acknowledgments

George Szasz, my brother and lifelong teacher and critic, helped to write and rewrite this book; Bill Whitehead, my editor at Doubleday, helped to give shape to it; and Margaret Bassett, my secretary, helped to bring it into being by continuing to protect my time and privacy and by her unfailing devotion, energy, and resourcefulness. I am deeply grateful to each of them.

"And the Lord said, 'Behold, they are one people, and they have all one language; and this is only the beginning of what they will do; and nothing that they propose to do will now be impossible for them. Come, let us go down, and there confuse their language, that they may not understand one another's speech.' . . . Therefore its name was called Babel, because there the Lord confused the language of all the earth. . . ."

GENESIS: 11:6–9

Contents

xi

Contents

Preface

We all know what is the first or "original" sin: "the knowledge of good and evil."

But we do not know, or tend to forget, what is the second sin: speaking clearly!

This is how the New English Bible describes it: "Once upon a time all the world spoke a single language and used the same words. As men journeyed in the east, they came upon a plain in the land of Shinar and settled there. They said to one another, 'Come, let us make bricks and bake them hard'; they used bricks for stone and bitumen for mortar. 'Come,' they said, 'let us build ourselves a city and a tower with its top in heaven, and make a name for ourselves; or we shall be dispersed all over the earth.' Then the Lord came down to see the city and tower which mortal men had built, and he said, 'Here they are, one people with a single language, and now they have started to do this; henceforward nothing they have a mind to do will be beyond their reach. Come, let us go down there and confuse their speech, so that they will not understand what they say to one another.' So the Lord dispersed them from there all over the earth, and they left off building the city. That is why it is called Babel, because the Lord there made a babble of the language of all of the world. . . ."[1]

This allegorical narrative—the parable of the second sin—displays the profoundest insight into the nature of man and, more particularly, into the nature of authority and its dependence on a monopoly over not only information but language itself: by expressing himself correctly, man becomes capable of rising to heaven, thus encroaching on God's territory. For this, God punishes man once more, by confusing his tongue.

Knowing and doing good and evil, thinking and speaking clearly—these are man's fundamental affronts against God, the child's against the parent, the citizen's against the state. This is why man is enjoined to avoid these sins; and why when he has committed them—as commit them he must if he is to be human—he has been punished by the Family, the Church, the State, and, in our day, by Psychiatry.

It seems to me that the second sin of Man, the sin of using language properly, and God's second punishment, the Divine Confusion, have been astonishingly neglected by students of man and language. Yet the importance and timelessness of the lesson this parable teaches are all too obvious. Authorities have always tended to honor and reward those who close man's mind by confusing his tongue, and have always tended to fear and punish those who open it by the plain and proper use of language. In so acting, authority has donned, successively, the mantle of Religion, of the State, and in our day, of Mental

[1] London: Oxford University Press and Cambridge University Press, 1970, p. 11.

Health or Psychiatry. But it matters not whether confusion and stupefaction are inspired divinely, governmentally, or psychiatrically—the result is the same: the parentification of authority and the infantilization of nearly everyone else.

It is against this process—an evil which authority always defines as a good—that many of the great polemicists and satirists of the West have fought. Pascal and La Rochefoucauld, Voltaire and Nietzsche, Bierce and Mencken are thus my models. My indebtedness to them for inspiring the form and style of the aphorisms, definitions, and maxims assembled here will, I hope, be evident to the reader and I hasten to acknowledge it.

Many of the entries refer to ideas or practices formally recognized as falling within the provinces of psychiatry and psychology. Others do not, unless one believes—as increasing numbers of people apparently believe—that everything people do is a legitimate matter for psychiatric inspection and management. I have tried to dispel this notion and other psychiatric mystifications, and to ridicule the psychiatric humbug that displaces ever more of our common sense and ordinary language.

THOMAS S. SZASZ

Syracuse, N.Y.
June 1, 1972

Introduction

Man is the animal that speaks. Understanding language is thus the key to understanding man; and the control of language, to the control of man.

Hence it is that men struggle not only over territory, food, and raw materials, but today perhaps most of all over language. For to control the Word is to be the Definer: God, king, pope, president, legislator, scientist, psychiatrist, madman—you and me. God defines everything and everyone. The totalitarian leader aspires to similar grandeur. The ordinary person defines some aspects of himself and of a few others. But even the most modest and powerless of men defines something no one else can: his own dreams.

And we are all defined, as well: by our genes which shape us; our parents who name us; our society which classifies us; and so on.

It has long seemed to me that some of the fundamental problems of psychiatry are really quite simple: they center around a struggle for definition between the so-called mental patient on the one side and his family, society, and psychiatrist on the other. Each party to this contest speaks a different language, whose content and consequences he tries to impose on his adversary. Although the contest sometimes looks like a debate, it is actually a bitter fight for survival, and, like all such struggles, it is decided not by logic but by power.

For example, the "patient" says he is Jesus; the psychiatrist says he is not Jesus, but a schizophrenic. The language of madness is thus one kind of jargon, and that of psychiatry another kind. In other words, some (though emphatically not all!) of the people who are called crazy abuse language; and so do many of the people who categorize and treat them psychiatrically. The result—whether it be schizophrenic claim called "symptom" or psychiatric counterclaim called "diagnosis"—is debased and dehumanized language.

Although languages have, as George Steiner observed, "great reserves of life," they are not inexhaustible: ". . . there comes a breaking point. Use a language to conceive, organize, and justify Belsen; use it to make out specifications for gas ovens; use it to dehumanize man during twelve years of calculated bestiality. Something will happen to it. . . . Something of the lies and sadism will settle in the marrow of the language."[1]

What in Steiner's view happened to the German language under the influence of Nazism applies, *mutatis mutandis,* but with even greater force, to what happens to ordinary language under the influence of psychiatry. Use language to conceive, organize, and justify the Salpêtrière, Burghölzli, and St. Elizabeths Hospital; use

[1] "The Hollow Miracle" (1959), in *Language and Silence: Essays on Language, Literature, and the Inhuman* (New York: Atheneum, 1967), p. 101.

it to make out specifications for chains and strait jackets, electroshock and frontal lobotomy; use it to dehumanize man during three hundred years of calculated bestiality, and something will happen to it. . . . Something of the lies and sadism will settle in the marrow of the language.

The abuse ordinary language has suffered at the hands of the madman *and* the mad-doctor has now lasted, not twelve years, like the Nazi regime, but nearly three hundred. And its end is nowhere in sight.

I have shown elsewhere[2] how, as a result of this process, neither the language of the mental patient nor that of the psychiatrist is serviceable for the proper description of either madness or our reactions to it. Each language is debased by systematic fraudulence, by the overwhelming effort on the part of the protagonist to impose his own image of the world on the other, and by justifying any means used to achieve this end.

To be sure, there are some who, perhaps because they believe that conventional wisdom is truth, refuse to question the language of psychiatry and see in it a key to the cure of mental illness. And there are others who, perhaps because they believe that the underdog is always right, glamorize and romanticize the language of madness and see in it a key to the proper understanding of the human dilemma.

To me, however, the choice between these two languages is a Hobson's choice. A dignified and humane understanding of man—his experiences and conflicts, his

---

[2] See, for example, *The Myth of Mental Illness: Foundations of a Theory of Personal Conduct* (New York: Hoeber-Harper, 1961), and *Ideology and Insanity: Essays on the Psychiatric Dehumanization of Man* (Garden City, N.Y.: Doubleday Anchor, 1970).

strengths and weaknesses, his saintliness and his bestiality —all this requires a rejection of the languages of both madness and mad-doctoring, and a fresh commitment to the conventional, disciplined, and artistic use of the language of the educated layman.

In short, I have here chosen to follow George Orwell's example. He stated the general problem—the medical and psychiatric dimensions of which are here my special concerns—in this way: "The great enemy of language is insincerity. When there is a gap between one's real and one's declared aims, one turns as it were instinctively to long words and exhausted idioms, like a cuttlefish squirting out ink. In our age there is no such a thing as 'keeping out of politics.' All issues are political issues, and politics itself is a mass of lies, evasions, folly, hatred, and schizophrenia."[3]

Since the power of all the professions that serve the public rests in large part on their loyal members' ability to confuse and thus dominate the public, it should not surprise us that not only the languages of medicine and psychiatry, but also those of education and law, are composed mainly of what Orwell called "ready-made phrases" whose function is to "anesthetize the brain."[4]

Orwell's remedy for all this lay in the Christian tradition that hopes and labors for the amelioration of great evils through small changes in the behavior of the single individual. "One . . . ought to recognize," he concluded, "that the present political chaos is connected with the

[3] "Politics and the English Language" (1946), in *The Orwell Reader: Fiction, Essays, and Reportage* (New York: Harcourt, Brace, Jovanovich, 1956), pp. 355–66; pp. 363–64.

[4] *Ibid.*, p. 364.

Introduction

decay of language, and that one can probably bring about some improvement by starting at the verbal end. If you simplify your English, you are freed from the worst follies of orthodoxy. You cannot speak any of the necessary dialects, and when you make a stupid remark its stupidity will be obvious, even to yourself. Political language . . . is designed to make lies sound truthful and murder respectable, and to give an appearance of solidity to pure wind. One cannot change this all in a moment, but one can at least change one's own habits. . . ."[5]

One can indeed, but only at the cost of willingly shouldering the burden of guilt incurred by committing not only the first but also the second sin.

[5] *Ibid.*, p. 366.

The Second Sin

Childhood

Childhood is a prison sentence of twenty-one years.

❋ ❋ ❋

To the child, control means care and love; to the adult, disdain and repression. Herein lies the fundamental dilemma and task of society: to encourage parents to love and control their children, and politicians to respect their fellow citizens and to leave them alone (except when the latter deprive others of life, liberty, or property).

Modern societies are well on their way to inverting this arrangement: They encourage parents to fake respect for their children and thus justify their failure to control them; and politicians to fake love for their fellow citizens and thus justify their efforts to exercise unlimited control over them.

❋ ❋ ❋

Permissiveness is the principle of treating children as if they were adults; and the tactic of making sure they never reach that stage.

❋ ❋ ❋

If a child is well treated, he may grow up to expect to get something for nothing; if ill treated, to have to give something for nothing. To steer a middle course between the Scylla of "psychopathy" and the Charybdis of "masochism" is the difficult task, first of the parent, and then of the developing child himself.

* * *

A child becomes an adult when he realizes that he has a right not only to be right but also to be wrong.

* * *

In the United States today there is a pervasive tendency to treat children like adults, and adults like children. We speak of infantilizing adults, and call their childish behavior infantilism. We should recognize the counterpart of this pattern: causing children to behave in an adultlike fashion, which results in "adulticism." The options of children are steadily expanded, while those of adults are progressively constricted.

In short, we treat fewer and fewer people as they really are. By allegedly protecting children from the evils of authoritarianism, and adults from the evils of competition, we define and maintain control over them, while claiming that we are helping them.

Family

In the modern family, the psychological problems of its members are not Oedipus and Electra complexes, but, more often, competitions for care, attention, and freedom. For example, in a family with young children, the father and the children often compete for the mother, and the mother might have to protect the children from the father's efforts to deprive them of maternal affection; whereas in a family with children on the verge of maturity, the mother and the children often compete for the father and the father might have to protect the children from the mother's efforts to infantilize them.

* * *

A mother (or father) says: "I wanted to give my children what I didn't have myself as a child." The upshot is that she exhausts herself in the effort, becomes envious of her own child, and ends by withdrawing and giving her child even less than her parents had given her.

The moral: consider yourself lucky if you take as good care of your children as your parents have of you. You might even do a little better, provided you don't aim too high.

Marriage

Marriage is a gift man gives to a woman for which she never forgives him.

* * *

The marriage certificate is proof of heterosexual normality. Many young people need it, to convince themselves and others that they are OK.

* * *

The most powerful contemporary symbol of the "sale" of women, and even more of their own "sellout," is not prostitution, nor the Playmate of the Month, nor any of the numerous discriminations women complain about; instead, I think it is the bridal section of the Sunday newspapers. This journalistic institution confirms and legitimates that just as the proper way for a child to be defined is through his association with his family of origin, so the proper way for a young woman to be defined is through her association with her husband-to-be.

* * *

Psychiatrists construct elaborate explanations for why people marry and divorce. But the meaning of these acts

5

is fairly self-evident. What requires explanation is why individuals stay married.

* * *

Marriage is a legally binding contract which the contracting parties are expected to make without legal assistance, but which they are prohibited by law from dissolving without such assistance.

* * *

Modern marriage is so difficult an arrangement because it is neither a truly contractual relationship nor a truly status relationship. Hence it is that neither husband nor wife can be sure exactly what each can expect of the other, and that both so often feel subjected to each other's whims. In short, contemporary marriage often combines the constraints of contract and the caprices of status.

* * *

If men and women about to be married were truly equal, why would they marry? Instead of a formal contract, an informal agreement would serve their purposes just as well. But since they are not equal, marriage now serves the bride to deceive the groom and vice versa: each thinks he or she will get the better of the bargain. Frequently, each soon concludes that he or she got the worst of it. In the language of game theory, then, contemporary marriage is often a negative-sum game: it is a game with two players both of whom can, and often do, lose simultaneously.

Modern marriage may, however, be a transitional stage, between the past arrangement, based on domination and subordination, which was a clear-cut zero-sum game—usually the man winning what the woman was losing; and a future arrangement, based on true economic and legal equality, which would be a clear-cut non-zero-sum game—each partner winning something as a result of the cooperation between them.

Love

We often speak of love when we really should be speaking of the drive to dominate or to master, so as to confirm ourselves as active agents, in control of our own destinies and worthy of respect from others.

* * *

Love is admiration or awe; compassion or pity. One might thus speak of the human tragedy of the improbability of love between equals. But perhaps the tragedy lies elsewhere, namely, in the spirit of modernity that has put love above dignity, the desire to be loved above the desire to be respected.

9

Sex

n human beings, sex is not so much an instinct as it is
, language, a signaling device. Being sexually desirable
typically for a woman) means: "He wants me, I *must*
»e worthwhile." Being sexually desirous (typically for a
nan) means: "I want her, I *must* know what life is for."

* * *

Vhat we consider to be normal sexuality is the result of
ge-old relations of domination and submission between
nen and women. This allocates certain rule-following
patterns to each sex; it also makes possible a certain num-
per of additional sexual roles through cross-identification
ind various tactics of rule rejection. Equality between
he sexes would mean that each person, and each sex,
pecomes the legitimate source of rules about how sexual
relations may be conducted. This would result in sexual
anomie, a condition many men and women find them-
elves in today. In this situation there are no fixed be-
avior patterns through which men may confirm them-
elves as men, and women as women. Not knowing what,
f any, rule to follow, individuals doubt the meaningful-
iess of any sexual role. They soon develop a longing for

11

sexual leaders; hence the popularity of Albert Ellis, David Reuben, Masters and Johnson.

* * *

Competence in heterosexuality, or at least the appearance or pretense of such competence, is as much a public affair as a private one. Thus, going steady is a high school diploma in heterosexuality; engagement a B.A.; marriage an M.A.; and children a Ph.D.

* * *

Masturbation: the primary sexual activity of mankind. In the nineteenth century, it was a disease; in the twentieth, it's a cure.

The preferred mode of sexual gratification for those who prefer the imaginary to the real.

* * *

Masturbation is more a matter of self-control than of self-love.

* * *

Perversion: sexual practice disapproved by the speaker.

* * *

The modern erotic ideal: man and woman in loving sexual embrace experiencing simultaneous orgasm through genital intercourse. This is a psychiatric-sexual myth useful for fostering feelings of sexual inadequacy and personal inferiority. It is also a rich source of "psychiatric patients."

* * *

One cannot be an individual, a person separate from others (family, society, etc.), without having secrets. It

because secrets separate people that individualists
easure them and collectivists condemn them.

As keeping secrets separates people, so sharing them
rings them together. Gossip, confessional, psychoanaly-
s, each involves communicating secrets and thus estab-
shing human relationships. Traditionally, sex has been a
ry private, secretive activity. Herein perhaps lies its
owerful force for uniting people in a strong bond. As
e make sex less secretive, we may rob it of its power to
old men and women together.

Women

It is more difficult for a woman, especially for an attractive woman, to live an independent and active life than it is for a man, because young women are easily diverted from the patient pursuit of competence by a premature, but inauthentic, pseudo-competence. It actually takes very little to perform the "service" of sexually satisfying a young man, but young women are generally "rewarded" for it through marriage and participation in the economic and social status of their husbands. When women later discover that they can do little, that they lack competence in many areas, and are, in a way, "good for nothing," it is too late. Indeed, the more intensely they realize and articulate their predicament, the more likely they are to be diagnosed as mentally ill—that is, as suffering from hysteria, depression, or schizophrenia; and the more loudly they complain of their predicament, the more likely they are to be psychiatrically punished for it—that is, by toxic chemicals, by involuntary mental hospitalization, and by electroshock and lobotomy.

*　*　*

The Second Sin

Like the Jews waiting for their Messiah, women wait for their man—each for her own "savior." Somewhere, deep in their hearts, women expect, hope against hope, for happiness with the "right" man, with the man whose love will give meaning to their lives. This expectancy—passive and yet demanding, patient and yet angry—is perhaps a characteristic expression of the oppressed person's basic life experience; that is, of a helplessness vis-à-vis the demands of life, together with a hopelessness to overcome it unaided by an all-powerful ally, a "savior."

* * *

There are two main reasons why women are unequal to men, and they are essentially the same as why some men are unequal to some other men. One is money: as a rule, men "make" it, whereas women "receive" it—from men, for domestic, sexual, or other services. The other is the significance of what they do: men "are busy" with "important" things, like politics and economics, science and technology, whereas women "keep busy" with "unimportant" things, like caring for children and shopping, cleaning and cooking. To the extent that women gain economic self-control (which is not the same as gaining wealth) and enhance the social significance of their daily activities, and to that extent alone, they will become men's equals—and superiors.

Ethics

Ethics: obsolete; superseded by the diagnosis and treatment of disease.

*   *   *

Good: obsolete; superseded by sane, mentally healthy, healthy.

*   *   *

Bad: obsolete; superseded by insane, mentally ill, sick.

*   *   *

There are only three major ethical modes of conduct.

1. The Golden Rule: doing unto others as we would want them to do unto us.

2. The Rule of Respect: doing unto others as they want us to do unto them.

3. The Rule of Paternalism: doing unto others as we, in our superior wisdom, know ought to be done unto them in their own best interests.

*   *   *

There are three major ethical systems, each identifiable by its object or symbol of ultimate value—God, the State, Man. The most grievous offense in each is not believing

17

in, not respecting, not taking seriously—God, the State
Man. In theism, the ultimate offense is atheism; in statism, it is anarchism; and in humanism, it is disbelief in
and disrespect of the individual, the person. It is a measure of how far we now are from a genuinely humanistic
ethic that not believing in human beings, not respecting
them, and not taking them seriously not only do not constitute grave offenses, but, on the contrary, are regarded
as virtuous achievements—namely, as signs of true belief
in "scientific socialism" in the East, and in "scientific
psychology and psychiatry" in the West.

*　*　*

Three R's: Reciprocity. Respect. Responsibility. The
three pillars of the ethics of autonomy.

*　*　*

Equality is inspiring as a legal ideal, stifling as a social
reality.

*　*　*

God is a metaphor of the Higher Law. For the atheist
man is the measure of all things. This leaves him with the
problem of: which man? The slave answers: the great
leader! The master answers: me! Both are wrong. Lest
human beings too easily justify themselves, there must be
a law above and beyond them. Few can accept this prop-
osition as an abstract principle; nearly everyone can
accept it when it is cast in the imagery of a deity.

*　*　*

In the *Inferno*, Dante assigns a fitting punishment to
those who, in their lives, were for neither good nor evil,
and to those who took no sides in the Rebellion of the

Angels. Confined forever in the Vestibule of Hell, Dante
describes them thus:

> "Sweet Spirit,
>
> what souls are these who run through this black haze?"
> And he [Virgil] to me: "These are the nearly soulless
> whose lives concluded neither blame nor praise.
>
> They are mixed here with that despicable corps
> of angels who were neither for God nor Satan, but
> only for themselves. The High Creator scourged them
> from Heaven for its perfect beauty, and Hell will
> not receive them since the wicked might feel some
> glory over them." And I:
>
> "Master, what gnaws at them so hideously their
> lamentation stuns the very air?" "They have no
> hope of death," he answered me,
>
> "and in their blind and unattaining state their
> miserable lives have sunk so low that they must
> envy every other fate. No word of them survives
> their living season. Mercy and Justice deny
> them even a name. Let us not speak of them:
> look, and pass on."[1]

In modern textbooks of psychiatry, the soulless men of
Dante come closest to those classified as mentally
healthy, all others, exhibiting passion for either good or
evil, being classified as suffering from one or another
form of mental illness.

[1] Dante Alighieri, *The Inferno,* a verse rendering for the modern
reader by John Ciardi (New York: Mentor, 1954), pp. 42–43.

Education

A teacher should have maximal authority, and minimal power.

* * *

In adult education there is an inverse relationship between power and learning. If the expert has too much power over the student, he ceases to be a teacher and becomes instead a leader or propagandist.

* * *

Every act of conscious learning requires the willingness to suffer an injury to one's self-esteem. That is why young children, before they are aware of their own self-importance, learn so easily; and why older persons, especially if vain or important, cannot learn at all.

Anatole France was right when he observed that: *"Les savants ne sont pas curieux."* ("The savants are not curious.") They can't afford to be: their lofty status depends on their knowing, and is undermined, or so they (and others) often feel, by their not knowing but trying to find out.

Pride and vanity can thus be greater obstacles to learning than stupidity. Psychoanalysis is an effort to teach the "patient" something about himself without humiliating him in the process; often, he could learn what the analyst teaches him from his wife (or husband), friends, children, or himself; but this would entail a loss of face which, he feels, he cannot afford.

Similarly, the person who cannot stop talking, who rambles on instead of listening, displays his fear of being found inadequate: he talks not to say something but to stop the other from exposing his weakness.

* * *

Compulsory education is the chink in the armor of capitalist societies: they try to teach children the values of contract and initiative, but base their educational system on compulsion and conformity. Communist societies suffer from no such inconsistency: they try to teach children the values of command and obedience, and their educational system is consistent with inculcating this ethic.

Language

It would seem likely that aboriginal man first vocalized idiosyncratically; that is, each man made noise rather than spoke a language. When two or more individuals adapted their noisemaking to a common pattern, language was born. Language may thus constitute the original social contract, out of which grew all the others.

* * *

Language separates men from other animals. It also reduces them to the level of animals—as in calling Jews "vermin" or policemen "pigs."

* * *

In the animal kingdom, the rule is, eat or be eaten; in the human kingdom, define or be defined.

* * *

Mystification is the principal semantic tool of the would-be leader; demystification, of the man who wants to be his own master. Rousseau, Marx, Freud mystified; Emerson, Mill, Adler demystified. It is perhaps one of the immutable tragedies of the human condition that while the demystifier influences individuals, the mystifier moves multitudes.

* * *

A Hungarian proverb warns: "Tell the truth, and you will get your head bashed in." Only in free and egalitarian situations can people be truthful. Because such situations are rare, speaking the truth is a luxury few people can afford.

* * *

We often call truths "brutal" and lies "white." If language mirrors the soul of man, this usage reflects the image of an aging Dorian Gray.

* * *

When we couch behavior in the language of religion, we legitimize it; when we couch it in the language of psychiatry, we illegitimize it.

We say that Catholics who do not eat meat on Fridays and Jews who do not eat pork at all are devoutly religious; we do not say that Catholics suffer from recurrent attacks of meat phobia, or that Jews are afflicted with a fixed phobia of pork.

On the other hand, we say that women who do not leave their homes suffer from agoraphobia and men who do not fly in airplanes suffer from a pathological fear of flying; we do not say that these men and women are devout cowards.

* * *

The struggle for definition is veritably the struggle for life itself. In the typical Western two men fight desperately for the possession of a gun that has been thrown to the ground: whoever reaches the weapon first, shoots and lives; his adversary is shot and dies. In ordinary life, the struggle is not for guns but for words: whoever first defines the situation is the victor; his adversary, the victim. For example, in the family, husband and wife, mother and child do not get along; who defines whom as troublesome or mentally sick? Or, in the apocryphal story about Emerson visiting Thoreau in jail; Emerson asks: "Henry, what are you doing over there?" Thoreau replies: "Ralph, what are you doing over there?" In short, he who first seizes the word imposes reality on the other: he who defines thus dominates and lives; and he who is defined is subjugated and may be killed.

* * *

To the institutional psychiatrist, lies are delusions. In abolishing the lie, he abolishes language; and in abolishing language, he abolishes—as C. S. Lewis warned that he would—man.

* * *

To concepts like suicide, homicide, and genocide, we should add "semanticide"—the murder of language. The deliberate (or quasi-deliberate) misuse of language through hidden metaphor and professional mystification, breaks the basic contract between people, namely the tacit agreement on the proper use of words. Thus it is that the "great" philosophers and politicians whose aim was to control man, from Rousseau to Stalin and Hitler, have preached and practiced semanticide; whereas those who have tried to set man free to be his own master, from

Emerson to Kraus and Orwell, have preached and practiced respect for language.

* * *

Definers (that is, persons who insist on defining others) are like pathogenic microorganisms: each invades, parasitizes, and often destroys his victim; and, in each case, those whose resistance is low are the most susceptible to attack. Hence, those whose immunological defenses are weak are most likely to contract infectious diseases; and those whose social defenses are weak—that is, the young and the old, the sick and the poor, and so forth—are most likely to contract invidious definitions of themselves.

* * *

"He who excuses himself, accuses himself," says a French proverb. In other words, he who speaks in the language of excuses—using disability, illness, mental illness, ignorance, poverty, or whatever as an excuse for not doing this or that—has lost half the battle for self-esteem before even beginning the fight for it.

* * *

The rhetoricians of race are not content with repudiating the oppression of the Negro but acclaim that "black is beautiful"; the rhetoricians of drugs are not content with rejecting false claims about the harmfulness of certain drugs but assert that toxic chemicals "expand the mind"; the rhetoricians of madness are not content with opposing the psychiatric violence inflicted on persons labeled mentally ill but claim that schizophrenia is not a "breakdown" but a "breakthrough." In short, ours is an age in which partial truths are tirelessly transformed into total falsehoods and then acclaimed as revolutionary revelations.

* * *

If the essence of conversion hysteria is that it is an indirect, ambiguous sort of communication, then professional jargon may be regarded as semantic hysteria. When a person speaks or writes in political, psychiatric, or sociological jargon, he expresses himself with a certain indirectness and ambiguity; and like the hysteric, he dramatizes what he says as something profound, although it may be trivial. This indirection also allows the speaker to express dangerous and forbidden ideas without fear of retribution by censor or colleagues. Compare the articles in contemporary psychoanalytic journals with Freud's early case histories; or sociological studies on war with Hemingway's stories. In short, if you want to learn about psychology or psychiatry, do not read psychology or psychiatry, but great literature, and especially biography. In the professional literature, for every sentence that clarifies (if, indeed, there are any such), there are two that obscure and mystify. Were a novelist or playwright to write like that, he would never get published.

* * *

Philosophy is, literally, the love of knowledge; phobosophy is the fear of it. There are obviously more "phobosophers" in the world than philosophers.

* * *

Medical mendacities:

The prevention of parenthood is called "planned parenthood."

Homicide by physicians is called "euthanasia."

Imprisonment by psychiatrists is called "mental hospitalization."

* * *

Quod licet Jovi, non licet bovi (What is permitted to Jove, is not permitted to the cow):

Policemen receive bribes; politicians receive campaign contributions.

Marijuana and heroin are sold by pushers; cigarettes and alcohol are sold by businessmen.

Mental patients who use the courts to regain their liberty are troublemakers; psychiatrists who use the courts to deprive patients of their liberty are therapists.

If General Motors sells cars, it's called advertising; if the National Institute of Mental Health sells psychiatry, it's called education; if a streetwalker sells sex, it's called soliciting; if a street urchin sells heroin, it's called pushing dope.

Classification

Most psychiatric riddles rest on an inarticulated problem of fitting an act, concept, or person into one or another category. What is a hysterically paralyzed arm: pretense or proof of the disease called "hysteria"? What is the assertion that one is Jesus: lie or delusion? The problems that lie behind the basic ideological and religious conflicts of mankind are of the same sort: Is the Negro chattel or man? Is Jesus man or God?

❋ ❋ ❋

Psychiatric diagnoses are stigmatizing labels phrased to resemble medical diagnoses and applied to persons whose behavior annoys or offends others. Those who suffer from and complain of their own behavior are usually classified as "neurotic"; those whose behavior makes others suffer, and about whom others complain, are usually classified as "psychotic."

❋ ❋ ❋

Psychiatric nosology (the classification of mental diseases): the language of loathing.

❋ ❋ ❋

The Second Sin

If you fake money, you are called a counterfeiter; if an official document, a forger; if an identity, a con man, psychopath, or schizophrenic; if illness, a hysteric; if cures, a quack; if speaking in a foreign language, a glossologist; and so forth. In each case, we must never forget that a person or group may accept as real what is actually fake, and reject as fake what is actually real.

Justification

We experience or generate certain feelings to justify our intended actions. For example, the young woman who wants to have intercourse with her boy friend: "I love him (*therefore* it's all right to go to bed with him)"; the young man who does not want to work for his father: "I hate him (*therefore* I can't work for him)." In short, affect legitimizes action.

* * *

What anxiety is to the timid, courage is to the brave: anxiety and courage are the motives and the justifications for either avoidance or engagement.

* * *

Man must justify his existence. To the question "What am I (good) for?" he offers a variety of replies, mainly depending on his age.

The child justifies himself by being obedient: "I am good. I please my parents."

The adolescent, by being promising: "I shall be important, successful, happy."

31

The young adult, by being sexual: "X is attracted to me. I give him (her) pleasure."

The adult, by being responsible: "My wife (husband), children, etc., need me. They could not manage without me."

The middle-aged person, by being powerful: "I control my wife (husband), children, colleagues, etc."

The old person, by being a survivor: "I have managed to hang on; I am still alive."

Each of these propositions confirms the importance of the individual in the world. Without such confirmation, the individual is likely to become ill, die, commit suicide, or suffer a "mental breakdown."

* * *

Man must justify his symbolic cannibalism, his victimization of others as acts of self-confirmation. In politics, the justification of victimization is supplied by the imagery of the "welfare of the people"; in domestic life, by "love"; in medicine, by "treatment."

* * *

Men are rewarded or punished not for what they do, but rather for how their acts are defined. This is why men are more interested in better justifying themselves than in better behaving themselves.

Significance

If man cannot bear a life of insignificance, and if a sense of significance is the same as a "religious outlook" on life, then mental health becomes a quest for significance. Jung understood this: "During the past thirty years, people from all the civilized countries have consulted me. . . . Among all my patients in the second half of life—that is to say, over thirty-five—there has not been one whose problem in the last resort was not that of finding a religious outlook on life. It is safe to say that every one of them fell ill because he had lost that which the living religions of every age have given to their followers, and none of them has been really healed who did not regain his religious outlook."[1]

Curiously, however, even Jung speaks of the people who consulted him with these problems as "ill." But it is precisely the technical idiom of medicine and psychiatry that stands in the way of recognizing and remedying these moral problems.

* * *

[1] Carl Gustav Jung, *Modern Man in Search of a Soul*, translated by W. S. Dell and C. F. Baynes (New York: Harcourt, Brace, Jovanovich, 1933), p. 229.

The central dramatic theme of life may be reduced to the following demand people make of each other: "Accept, validate, and reinforce my fantasy about myself! If you don't, I won't love you, I'll punish you, I'll leave you, I'll kill you." In short: "Authenticate me, or else!"

* * *

In many people's lives, the need for attention is the dominant motive. This explains why people often espouse one opinion one time, and its opposite soon after: it does not matter what they say, so long as it draws attention to them. Tolstoy was a dramatic example.

In his biography of Tolstoy, Henri Troyat remarks that Tolstoy's family and friends ". . . could not understand how he had married an upperclass girl after declaring that 'to marry a woman of society is to swallow the whole poison of civilization.'"

Psychoanalysts interpret this sort of behavior as the expression of ambivalence. Moralists call it hypocrisy. It may be both of these things. But it often is simply the result of a passion for attention, which cannot be as easily satisfied through consistent behavior.

* * *

What psychiatrists call "delusion of grandeur" is the assumption of an identity superior to the person's real identity, stubbornly claimed by the impersonator and equally stubbornly repudiated by those about him. Rejection of this kind of impersonation is often couched in the language of psychiatry, by calling the impersonator "delusional" and "psychotic," thus concealing the bitter conflict between his claims and the counterclaims of others behind a diagnostic label.

* * *

What psychiatrists call "delusion of persecution" is one of the most dramatic human defenses against the feeling of personal insignificance and worthlessness. In fact, no one cares a hoot about Jones. He is an extra on the stage of life. But he wants to be a star. He cannot become one by making a fortune on the stock market, or by getting a Nobel prize. So he claims that the FBI or the Communists are watching his every move, are tapping his phone, etc. Why would they be doing this, unless Jones were an enormously important person? In short, the paranoid delusion is a *problem* to the patient's family, employer, and friends; to the patient, it is a *solution* to the problem of the meaning(lessness) of his life.

* * *

The psychotic (and especially the paranoid schizophrenic) defines society by the arrogant creation of meaning for himself, flagrantly disregarding society's conventions for doing so. For example, he declares that he is Jesus or that the Communists are persecuting him. This makes everyone around him secretly envious: how can his life be so interesting and important when theirs are so dull and unimportant? Secure in their conviction that the patient does not deserve the meaning he attributes to himself, they punish him by demeaning him: they define his claim as a delusion, declare him crazy, and treat him as the most unworthy of persons.

* * *

In many social situations there is now a disorderly shoving on the stage of life—as each person tries to push the others off stage and himself into the lead. Who is the "star" in the family: father, mother, or child? In the school: teacher or student? In the courtroom: defendant, bench, or bar? And there are new fashions for gaining stardom: prohibiting the taking of drugs and taking prohibited drugs; hijacking airplanes; making extravagant claims—for the effects of LSD, sexual fulfillment, racial conflict and integration, disarmament, the prevalence and dangers of mental illness, etc.

* * *

Negation is one of the most basic ways by which man creates meaning. If authority asserts that "X is good," the assertion that "X is bad" (or that "anti-X is good") becomes an immediate possibility for affirming one's identity and even one's superiority. Sexual pleasure, eating, making war on one's enemies have been ancient, pre-Christian values. They have generated ferocious commitments to chastity, self-starvation, and pacifism (as in early Christians, in Gandhi, etc.). Similarly, in our day, if authority is seen as sexually inhibited, youth proclaims sexual disinhibition as a transcendent value. The same affirmation of value by negation may be seen in such reversals as clean-dirty; rich-poor; competitive-noncompetitive; cleanshaven-bearded; shorthaired-longhaired.

* * *

An adolescent boy, neither bright nor industrious, repressed and put down at home, engages in a violent crime for which he is certain to be apprehended. Why does he do it? Because he feels that he is a "nothing," that he does not exist except as an object of abuse and derision. After his arrest, he becomes an actor in a significant drama: through his "responsibility" for the crime, he is reborn, he comes into existence, as a person. Later, while still a minor, he plans to marry, although this only promises to add to his still heavy burdens. I ask him why (he wants to marry the young woman who is already the mother of his child). He replies: "Because then I will at least be responsible for a wife and a child." Some people can give meaning to their lives by achievements in art and science, finance and politics; others, by assuming responsibilities for "dependents," wives or husbands, children or patients; and those who are unable or unwilling to follow either of these paths can give their lives meaning by violating the criminal or mental hygiene laws and thus assuming responsibility for their status as criminals or victims, madmen or misunderstood geniuses.

* * *

The proverb admonishes not to curse the darkness, but to light a candle. This seemingly good advice overlooks the advantages of cursing the darkness and not lighting a candle—namely, the cheaply earned self-esteem that comes from righteous indignation and seeing oneself as a victim; and the avoidance of facing the problem of what to do after one has lit the candle. Herein lie the benefits to the "patients" of the so-called severe mental diseases: while these "diseases" seem like problems to the psychiatrist, they are solutions—of the type that cursing the darkness is—to the "patients."

Emotions

Boredom is the feeling that everything is a waste of time; serenity, that nothing is.

* * *

Happiness is an imaginary condition, formerly often attributed by the living to the dead, now usually attributed by adults to children, and by children to adults.

* * *

Anxiety is the unwillingness to play even when you know the odds are for you.

Courage is the willingness to play even when you know the odds are against you.

* * *

Gratitude is contingent on feelings of equality or superiority. Men thus feel grateful not so much because others have treated them well (albeit this is usually a prerequisite for feeling grateful), but rather because they have equaled or surpassed their former benefactor. The moral: expect gratitude only from those who, whether through your help or their own efforts, have equaled or surpassed you in life.

Freedom

Men love liberty because it protects them from control and humiliation by others, and thus affords them the possibility of dignity. They loathe liberty because it throws them back on their own abilities and resources, and thus confronts them with the possibility of insignificance.

* * *

Freedom is what most people want for themselves, and what they most want to deprive others of.

* * *

When the psychiatrist approves of a person's actions, he judges that person to have acted with "free choice"; when he disapproves, he judges him to have acted without "free choice." It is small wonder that people find "free choice" a confusing idea: It looks as if "free choice" were a part of what a person being judged (often called "patient") *does,* whereas it is actually a part of what the person making the judgment (often called "psychiatrist") *thinks.*

Law

The state cannot "legalize" any act; it can only "criminalize" acts or leave them alone.

* * *

The fact that Americans speak about "legalizing" abortion, gambling, marijuana, and so forth shows that they no longer look down on their government as their servant but look up to it as their master. For to legalize is to permit; and to permit implies a relationship between a superior and a subordinate—as when a parent permits a child to go swimming, stay up late at night, or eat sweets after finishing his meal.

* * *

Traditional justice is based on the concepts of right and wrong; modern justice, on those of mental health and illness. When Solomon was confronted with two women both of whom claimed to be the mother of the same child, he talked to them and had them talk to him, and he awarded the child to the woman who, he inferred from the information he obtained, was the real mother. A modern American judge would proceed quite differently.

Concluding from the conflicting claims that one of the women must be "deluded" in believing that she is the mother, he would have both women examined by psychiatrists. The psychiatrists would then discover that one of the women was a fanatic, insisting that she wants the whole child or nothing, whereas the other is reasonable, willing to make a compromise and accept half a child; accordingly, they would declare the real mother to be suffering from schizophrenia, and would recommend awarding the child to the impostor—a recommendation the judge, respectful of the findings of medical experts—would rubber-stamp.

* * *

Formerly, Americans charged with murder were considered innocent until proven guilty; now they are considered insane until proven sane.

* * *

Psychiatric expert testimony: mendacity masquerading as medicine.

* * *

Judges and prosecutors, lawyers and psychiatrists, all protest their passionate desire to know why a person accused of a crime did what he did. But their actions completely belie their words: their efforts are now directed toward letting everyone speak in court but the defendant himself—especially if he is accused of a political or psychiatric crime.

* * *

An old adage (whose source I cannot locate) cautions the would-be lawmaker not to prohibit what he cannot enforce. For some time now, American lawmakers have followed the opposite rule—namely, that what they cannot control, they can at least prohibit.

* * *

Americans are still free to buy loaded guns, but are no longer free to buy empty syringes. These facts symbolize, perhaps better than any others, how far the American government has gone in abandoning the task of protecting safety, and in assuming the task of invading privacy.

* * *

Mental hygiene laws possess the most fearsome qualities of both civil and criminal laws: They are like civil laws in that they are not subject to constitutional limitations; and like criminal laws in that among their *de facto* penalties are deprivation of life, liberty, and property.

Punishment

If he who breaks the law is not punished, he who obeys
it is cheated. This, and this alone, is why lawbreakers
ought to be punished: to authenticate as good, and to
encourage as useful, law-abiding behavior.

The aim of the criminal law cannot be correction or
deterrence; it can only be the maintenance of the legal
order.

* * *

Punishment is no longer fashionable. Why? Because—
with its corollary, reward—it makes some people guilty
and others innocent, some good and others evil; in short,
it creates moral distinctions among men, and, to the
"democratic" mentality, this is odious. Our age seems to
prefer a meaningless collective guilt to a meaningful individual responsibility.

* * *

There can be no humane penology so long as punishment
masquerades as "correction." No person or group has the
right to "correct" a human being; only God does. But
persons and groups have the right to protect themselves

through sanctions that are, and should be called, "punishments," which, of course, may be as mild as a scolding or a small fine, or as severe as life imprisonment or death.

Control and Self-control

The goal of deception is the control and annihilation of the other; the result of self-deception is the loss of control and annihilation of the self.

* * *

"To believe your own thought" observed Emerson, "to believe that what is true for you in your private heart is true for all men—that is genius." But to impose what you believe is true for you upon all men, indeed upon a single individual—that is despotism.

* * *

In working, we generally exert control over some thing or person. When we hunt or fish, plow or reap, we control things. When we feed a baby, operate on a sick patient, or judge a criminal, we control a person. However, in complex, materially advanced societies, there are many situations that call for neither of these postures, but, on the contrary, require that we control ourselves and re-linquish a measure of control over ourselves to others, usually in exchange for money. This is especially true of professional work.

The Second Sin

Prostitution is said to be the world's oldest *profession*. It is, indeed, a model of all professional work: the worker relinquishes control over himself (herself), his (her) body—usually in a particular, clearly defined manner—in exchange for money. Because of the passivity it entails, this is a difficult and, for many, a distasteful, role.

* * *

The proverb warns that "You should not bite the hand that feeds you." But maybe you should, if it prevents you from feeding yourself.

* * *

Addiction, obesity, starvation (anorexia nervosa) are political problems, not psychiatric: each condenses and expresses a contest between the individual and some other person or persons in his environment over the control of the individual's body.

* * *

Every benefactor wants to be in control of his charge. The priest controls in the name of God; the physician, in the name of health. This universal propensity to control others conflicts with and contradicts the aim of making man a self-responsible individual.

* * *

Reciprocity: the mirage beckoning to mankind wandering in the desert of domination-submission.

* * *

Cooperation is contingent on mutual interdependence. An excess of both control and self-control is inimical to social cohesion. Too much control results in oppression and leads to noncooperation through rebellion. Too much self-control results in personal autarchy and leads to noncooperation through isolation. The delicate balance between control and self-control that social life requires is one of the reasons why tragedy is inherent in human existence.

* * *

Most people want self-determination for themselves and subjection for others; some want subjection for everyone; only a few want self-determination for everyone.

* * *

If someone does something we disapprove of, we regard him as bad if we believe we can deter him from persisting in his conduct, but we regard him as mad if we believe we cannot. In either case, the crucial issue is our control of the other: the more we lose control over him, and the more he assumes control over himself, the more, in case of conflict, we are likely to consider him mad rather than just bad.

* * *

A madman is one who has, or is alleged to have, lost control of himself. Psychiatry supplies the justification for controlling him. The person securely in control of himself frustrates others from controlling him; hence he is the object of both admiration and envy, awe and hate.

Personal Conduct

Men often treat others worse than they treat themselves, but they rarely treat anyone better. It is the height of folly to expect consideration and decency from a person who mistreats himself.

* * *

We pay too much attention to learning how to acquire habits, and too little to how to break them.

* * *

Knowledge is gained by learning; trust by doubt; skill by practice; and love by love.

* * *

The quality of our life depends largely on concordance or discordance between our desires and our duties.

If we can define and experience our duty as our desire—then we are happy, well-adjusted, normal. If this congruence breaks down, we feel cheated, frustrated, depressed; we may even go mad with rage toward, and envy of, those who were more selfish, and hence less dutiful, than we have been.

If we can define and experience our desire as our duty

—then our happiness or the lack of it shall depend on whether we can persuade others that such is indeed the case. In proportion as we succeed in persuading them, we become accredited as moral leaders: Tolstoy and Gandhi were eminently successful at this. In proportion as we fail in persuading them, we become defined as mad fanatics: the schizophrenic who kills and tries to get away with it, by claiming that God commanded him to do it, is an example; the discredited leader of an unsuccessful political revolution is another. If this congruence between our desire and duty breaks down and we recognize that what we thought was duty was merely desire, then we may go mad with guilt: our conscience will then haunt us and we may commit suicide in an effort to pay for our misdeeds and restore the inner balance between our desires and duties.

* * *

It is easier to do one's duty to others than to one's self. If you do your duty to others, you are considered reliable. If you do your duty to yourself, you are considered selfish.

* * *

Men are often afraid to rock the boat in which they hope to drift safely through life's currents, when, actually, the boat is stuck on a sandbar. They would be better off to rock the boat and try to shake it loose, or, better still, jump in the water and swim for the shore.

* * *

The phrase "self-made man" is typically nineteenth-century American. Elsewhere and before then, God made men; and since then, in all cultures, man has been made by societies, parents, genes, and environments. In short, today everyone and everything is credited and blamed for what a person is, except the person himself. This is ironic, since man now has more opportunities for creating himself than he has ever had in the past.

* * *

People often say that this or that person has not yet found himself. But the self is not something one finds; it is something one creates.

* * *

As the internal-combustion engine runs on gasoline, so the person runs on self-esteem: if he is full of it, he is good for a long run; if he is partly filled, he will soon need to be refueled; and if he is empty, he will come to a stop.

* * *

Man cannot long survive without air, water, and sleep. Next in importance comes food. And close on its heels, solitude.

* * *

Solitary confinement is a severe punishment because people need other people. But people also need to be alone. For many persons, having to be with others is much more painful than having to be alone.

* * *

Clear thinking requires courage rather than intelligence.

* * *

The Second Sin

"Where there is a will, there is a way," says the proverb. Not entirely true; but it is true that where there is no will, there is no way.

*　*　*

It is generally believed that activity and mastery are virtually synonymous. To learn to walk, swim, drive a car, and so forth, all require active mastery of our bodies or environment. But certain kinds of achievement require a kind of controlled passivity, a mastery of our fear of passivity and helplessness. Among these the following are of interest:

Sex. Pleasurable sexual intercourse with a partner who is one's equal or superior is possible only if, and in proportion as, one accepts one's need to be passive. Masturbation and the use of prostitutes remain favored because they make possible a wholly "active," self-controlled sexual performance.

Learning. The person who cannot accept his ignorance cannot learn. Inventiveness and creativity depend on the individual's ability to let himself sink deeply into a feeling of mystery, to be overcome later by proportional efforts at mastery. Imitation of others and reliance on accepted authorities are time-honored and popular because they make possible a wholly "active," self-controlled intellectual performance.

Illness and death. To be ill and die properly one must be passive. Hypochondriasis and suicide offer alternatives in substituting activity for passivity, mastery (or the illusion of it) for helplessness (or the fear of it). More generally, we achieve "active" mastery over illness and death by delegating all responsibility for their management to physicians, and by exiling the sick and the dying to hospitals. But hospitals serve the convenience of staff not patients: we cannot be properly ill in a hospital, nor die in one decently; we can do so only among those who love and value us. The result is the institutionalized dehumanization of the ill, characteristic of our age.

*   *   *

The stupid neither forgive nor forget; the naïve forgive and forget; the wise forgive but do not forget.

*   *   *

Conscience: made out of reasonable expectations; soluble in alcohol; destroyed by bureaucracies and other types of collectives.

Social Relations

person cannot make another happy, but he can make
m unhappy. This is the main reason why there is more
1happiness than happiness in the world.

       ✻   ✻   ✻

key concept for understanding behavior (both "nor-
al" and "abnormal") is impersonation. There are two
asic kinds of impersonations: those that are publicly
pported and legitimated, and those that are not. Ex-
nples of the former are an actor playing a part in a play
* a small boy playing fireman. Examples of the latter are
healthy housewife complaining of aches and pains or
unemployed carpenter claiming that he is Jesus.
'hen persons stubbornly cling to and aggressively pro-
aim publicly unsupported role definitions, they are
lled psychotic.

       ✻   ✻   ✻

very human encounter validates or invalidates some or
l of the participants in it. None is neutral.
In the "helping professions," particularly in institu-
nal psychiatry and social work, each encounter typi-

cally validates the professional (as giving something of value) and invalidates the client (as receiving something of value). In business transactions, each encounter typically validates both parties (as each having to offer something of value). When close affectional relations such as marriage and friendship come to grief, each encounter typically invalidates both parties (as each being injurious to the other).

* * *

Human relations are problematic because men are driven by opposing but often equally powerful needs and passions, especially the needs for security and freedom. To satisfy the need for security, people seek closeness and commitment, and the more they attain these, the more oppressed they feel. To satisfy their need for freedom, people seek independence and detachment, and the more they attain these, the more isolated they feel. And in all such things, the wise pursue the golden mean; and the lucky attain it.

* * *

Mysticism joins and unites; reason divides and separates. People generally crave belonging more than understanding. Hence the prominent role of mysticism, and the limited role of reason, in human affairs.

* * *

To whom does a person's body belong? Does it belong to his parents, as it did, to a very large extent, when he was a child? Or to the state? Or to the sovereign? Or to God? Or, finally, to himself? Countless moral and

Social Relations

sychiatric controversies—about abortion, contraception, rugs, sex, and suicide—revolve around inexplicit and unlarified premises about this question.

* * *

Nietzsche defined man as the "animal that is able to make romises. . . ."[1] I would add that he is also the animal r being that is able to—indeed, that loves to—break romises. In short, man is a liar—with a limitless capacy for deceiving himself and for being deceived by thers.

* * *

Equality in human relations is like the ideal gas of the hysicist: a model impossible of actual realization. One nust be definer or defined; one cannot be neither or oth. The most, then, that can be expected of human relations is a mutually satisfying reciprocity of role, an arrangement not necessarily facilitated by strivings for quality.

* * *

Power corrupts. But so does powerlessness. Respect for uman dignity requires a wide distribution of power; in ther words, the moderation of one man's power by that f another. Limited power is thus a necessary, but not a ufficient, condition for the flowering of respect for self nd others. The additional requirement for it is the love f justice.

* * *

[1] Quoted by Harold C. Havighurst, *The Nature of Private Contract* (Evanston, Ill.: Northwestern University Press, 1961), p. 12.

The Second Sin

Adulthood is the ever-shrinking period between childhood and old age. It is the apparent aim of modern industrial societies to reduce this period to a minimum.

* * *

Adults often define submission to authority as a sign of
being grown-up. For example, a father tells his son who
is reluctant to go to school or to the dentist: "Act like a
man!" What he actually means is that he wants his son
to act like an obedient child.

Men and women often fail to discriminate between
when they ought to or want to comply with authority
and when they ought to or want to resist its demands. In
Nazi Germany, Jews and gentiles alike acted vis-à-vis
Nazi authority like the "good soldiers" little boys are
told to act like. Patients and physicians in both Communist and capitalist societies now act with the same
childish submissiveness toward the demands of the state
couched in the rhetoric of illness and health care.

In short, indiscriminate submission to authority and
indiscriminate resistance to it are both childish. The mature person is characterized by his ability to decide, according to morally significant criteria, when to cooperate
with authority and when not to.

* * *

Keeping another person waiting is a basic tactic for
defining him as inferior and oneself as superior. When
women are courted, they keep the men waiting; after
marriage, husbands keep their wives waiting. In the end
we are all kept waiting, and we all hate it! How men
hate waiting while their wives shop for clothes and

trinkets; how women hate waiting, often for much of their lives, while their husbands shop for fame and glory.

* * *

Self-respect is to the soul as oxygen is to the body. Deprive a person of oxygen, and you kill his body; deprive him of self-respect, and you kill his spirit. Hence it is that the wise treat self-respect as nonnegotiable, and will not trade it for health or wealth or anything else; whereas the foolish will trade it, only to discover too late that it does not profit a man to gain the whole world if it costs him his self-respect.

* * *

Intolerant persons reject those who are unlike themselves; tolerant persons accept them—provided they become like themselves. This is why children are usually accepted only as potential adults; sick patients only as potentially healthy persons; Jews only as potential Christians; and so forth.

* * *

Man appears unable or unwilling to accept the reality of human conflict. It is never simply man who offends against his fellow man. Someone or something—the devil, masturbation, mental illness—always intervenes, to obscure, excuse, and explain away man's terrifying inhumanity to man.

* * *

There are two kinds of leadership: for dependence and for independence. Historically, the only kind of readily recognizable and publicly visible leadership has been leadership for dependence on authority. When such leadership is successful, it results in the recruitment of faithful followers who, through their claims and conduct confirm the glory and verify the wisdom of the "great leader." In contrast, leadership for independence is of low visibility and hence difficult to recognize. When such leadership is successful, it results not in faithful followers but in independent individuals who, through their claims and conduct, confirm only their own authenticity.

* * *

What does man do with his fellow man who has fallen behind in the race of life? The liberal puts money in his pocket and a social worker on his back. Who among us really tries to put him on his feet so he can run again and perhaps even surpass us? When is the helpless really helped, the weak strengthened? And when is helpfulness merely a strategy for confirming the helper in his role as priest, physician, philanthropist?

* * *

When people speak about the dehumanizing treatment accorded to some groups—especially the aged, the mentally retarded, and the mentally ill—they often emphasize their disapproval by asserting that these persons are treated like animals. But that is quite false. People almost never treat animals as badly as they do other people. And they never systematically so mistreat them.

The reason is obvious: it lies not in man's viciousness but in his reasonableness. Animals—for example, dogs, cattle, or chickens—are useful to man, who has therefore good reason to treat them reasonably well. When such animals have served their usefulness, man kills them and has therefore again no reason to mistreat them. And animals—especially domestic animals—are readily controlled, more readily than people; hence, again, there is no need to mistreat them.

On the other hand, the individuals (and groups) most mistreated by people are those who do not meet any of the above criteria: the aged, the mentally retarded, and the mentally sick are not useful; cannot be easily controlled; and cannot be killed. Their very existence is thus experienced as a burden by all those on whom they depend and who take care of them, and who therefore retaliate by inflicting on them a fate not only worse than death, but far worse than any inflicted on animals.

* * *

The many faces of intimacy: the Victorians could experience it through correspondence, but not through cohabitation; contemporary men and women can experience it through fornication, but not through friendship.

* * *

Beware of people who don't know how to say "I am sorry." They are weak and frightened, and will, sometimes at the slightest provocation, fight with the desperate ferocity of a frightened animal that feels cornered.

* * *

Two wrongs don't make a right, but they make a good excuse.

* * *

When a person can no longer laugh at himself, it is time for others to laugh at him.

Medicine

Control in the medical relationship is subtly defined and symbolized by the territory on which it occurs (and which depends in part on who pays for the service): when in the patient's home, the patient is in control; when in the physician's office, the physician is in control; and when in the hospital, Medical Authority or the state is in control. When medical practice was in the free marketplace (as it had been during the nineteenth century), the rich were seen in their homes and the poor in charity hospitals; when it came under the domination of the medical profession (during the first half of the twentieth century, in the United States), the rich were seen in physicians' offices and the poor in public clinics of various sorts; and when it came under the domination of the state (since the end of World War II), the center of gravity of medical practice shifted increasingly toward the hospital, rich and poor, patient and physician, all losing control to medical administrators and government bureaucrats. This may in part explain why, although physicians can now do more for their patients than ever before, both patients and doctors are more than ever dissatisfied with medicine.

* * *

In business, where monopolies are no longer the danger they once were, we zealously guard ourselves against them. In the professions, where monopolies are an immense danger, we mindlessly clamor for enlarging their scope and power.

In business, the seller advertises and competes with other entrepreneurs, and the buyer has a wide choice of products and services. In medicine, the physician cannot advertise and does not compete with other doctors, and the patient has a correspondingly narrow choice of products and services.

Yet we wonder what's wrong with the "delivery" of medical care, and redouble our efforts to transform medicine into a government-controlled monopoly.

* * *

The greatest analgesic, soporific, stimulant, tranquilizer, narcotic, and to some extent even antibiotic—in short, the closest thing to a genuine panacea—known to medical science is work.

* * *

Idiopathic: medical jargon for "We don't know what it is, what causes it, or what to do for it—but we won't admit any of this to laymen or patients."

* * *

Reassurance: a type of medical mendacity, consisting of the physician communicating calculated falsehoods to the patient which the physician claims the patient wants to hear.

* * *

Treatment: 1. Intervention sought by patient from physician for the amelioration or cure of disease. 2. Punishment (as in "Let's give him the treatment . . ."); especially popular in psychiatric institutions and totalitarian countries. 3. Anything, usually of an unpleasant nature, that we want to do to another person. Often confused with what our unfeeling ancestors called "punishment," but which, thanks to the discoveries of modern psychiatry, we now realize are forms of medical treatment.

* * *

The concept of "treatment" is the grand legitimizer of our age. Call whatever you want to do "treatment," and you are instantly hailed as a great humanitarian and scientist. Freud decided to listen and talk to people, so he called conversation "therapy" and psychoanalysis is now recognized as a form of medical treatment. Cerletti decided to give people electrical convulsions, so he called electroshock "therapy" and it is now recognized as a form of medical treatment. Masters decided to train men to perform sexually, so he called procuring prostitutes for them "therapy" and pimping became a novel form of medical treatment.

* * *

When a person eats too much, his intestines are short-circuited: this is called a "bypass operation for obesity." When a person thinks too much, his brain is short-circuited: this is called "frontal lobotomy for schizo-phrenia."

* * *

The final medical solution to human problems: remove everything from the body that is diseased or protesting, leaving only enough organs which—by themselves, or hooked up to appropriate machines—still justify calling what is left of the person a "case"; and call the procedure "humanectomy."

Drugs

No drug can expand consciousness; the only thing a drug can expand is the earnings of the company that makes it.

* * *

Voltaire said: "I disapprove of what you say, but I will defend to the death your right to say it." But who will say today: "I disapprove of what you take, but I will defend to the death your right to take it"? Yet it would seem to me that the right to take things is more elementary than the right to say things; for taking things is less likely to harm others than saying them. In a free society, it is none of the government's business what idea a man puts into his head; it should also be none of its business what drug he puts into his body.

* * *

Marx said that religion was the opiate of the people. In the United States today, opiates are the religion of the people.

* * *

The Nazis spoke of having a Jewish problem. We now speak of having a drug-abuse problem. Actually, "Jewish problem" was the name the Germans gave to the persecution of the Jews; "drug-abuse problem" is the name we give to the persecution of people who use certain drugs.

* * *

The narcotics laws are our dietary laws. Since this is the age of science, not religion, psychiatrists are our rabbis, heroin is our pork, and the addict is our unclean person.

* * *

Treating addiction to heroin with methadone is like treating addiction to scotch with bourbon.

* * *

Powerful "addictions"—whether to smoking cigarettes or injecting heroin—are actually both very difficult and very easy to overcome. Some people struggle vainly against such a habit for decades; others "decide" to stop and are done with it; and sometimes those who have long struggled in vain manage suddenly to rid themselves of the habit. How can we account for this? Not only is the pharmacology of the so-called addictive substance irrelevant to this riddle, but so is the personality of the so-called addict. What is relevant is whether "the addiction"—smoking, drinking, shooting heroin—is or is not a part of an internally significant dramatic production in which the "patient-victim" is the star. So long as it is (and if it is, the struggle to combat the addiction is only a part of the play), the person will find it difficult or impossible to give up his habit; whereas once he has decided to close down this play and leave the stage, he will find the grip of the habit broken and will "cure" himself of the "addiction" with surprising ease.

* * *

Some advocate that heroin be prohibited; others, that it be given "free" to "addicts." Both positions reveal a shocking lack of a sense of equity: Why should heroin be prohibited when alcohol and nicotine are not? Why should heroin be dispensed at the taxpayer's expense to those who crave it when alcoholic beverages and cigarettes are not to those who crave them? Furthermore, it is revealing of our propensity for meddling that every conceivable intervention in the lives of "addicts" is now seriously advocated and widely supported, save one: repealing all anti-drug laws and leaving so-called addicts alone.

* * *

Ours is truly an age of materialism. I say this not because we are fond of money or gadgets, but because we fear material threats more acutely than spiritual ones. Indeed, we deny spiritual things the power they have, and endow material things with an influence they do not have. We thus speak of a person being "under the influence" of alcohol, or heroin, or amphetamine, and believe that these substances affect him so profoundly as to render him utterly helpless in their grip. We thus consider it scientifically justified to take the most stringent precautions against these things and often prohibit their nonmedical, or even their medical, use. But a person may be under the influence not only of material substances but also of spiritual ideas and sentiments, such as patriotism, Catholicism, or Communism. But we are not afraid of these influences and believe that each person is, or ought to be, capable of fending for himself in a free marketplace of ideas. Herein precisely lies our moral turpitude: that we show more respect for drugs than for ideas.

Suicide

Suicide is a fundamental human right. This does not mean that it is morally desirable. It only means that society does not have the moral right to interfere, by force, with a person's decision to commit this act.

* * *

To prohibit what one cannot enforce is to degrade both authority and obedience, thus undermining not only respect for law, but respect for decency. To prohibit suicide is thus the ultimate folly, and the ultimate indecency.

* * *

He who does not accept and respect those who want to reject life does not truly accept and respect life itself.

* * *

The physician has unrestricted access to the modern pharmacological technology of suicide. Why shouldn't everyone else have the same "right" to kill himself easily, painlessly, and surely?

* * *

Doctors try to save lives; suicides try to throw them away. It is hardly surprising that the two get along so poorly. Like misers and spendthrifts, all they have in common is their differences.

❋ ❋ ❋

"Attempted suicide" is strategic psychiatric rhetoric; in most cases "attempted suicide" is actually "pretended suicide."

❋ ❋ ❋

Abortion is called "murder" or "feticide" by those who disapprove of it; and "birth control" by those who approve of it or who do not condemn it. Similarly, causing one's own death should be called "suicide" only by those who disapprove of it; and should be called "death control" by those who approve of it—or at least do not condemn it.

Psychiatry

There are two kinds of psychiatry: voluntary and involuntary, or contractual and institutional. To confuse these is like confusing friend and foe, truth and falsehood, freedom and slavery, life and death. Contractual psychiatry comprises all psychiatric interventions secured for themselves by persons prompted by their own personal difficulties or suffering. These interventions are characterized by the retention of complete control by the client over his relationship with the expert. The most important economic characteristic of contractual psychiatry is that the contractual psychiatrist is a private entrepreneur, paid for his services by his client. Its most important social characteristic is the avoidance of force and fraud (with legal penalties for their use), and reliance instead on a clear contractual agreement between client and expert. (See also Institutional Psychiatry.)

*　*　*

Psychiatry is a moral and social enterprise. The psychiatrist deals with problems of human conduct. He is, therefore, drawn into situations of conflict—often between the individual and the group. If we wish to understand psychiatry, we cannot avert our eyes from this dilemma: we must know whose side the psychiatrist takes—the individual's or the group's.

* * *

In general, those who pay for a psychiatric service are its beneficiaries; when people receive a psychiatric service without paying for it, they are the victims, not the beneficiaries, of psychiatry.

* * *

Much of what now passes as mental illness is actually force and fraud—the so-called patient trying to coerce others by pretending to be sick. Similarly, much of what now passes as psychiatry is also force and fraud—the so-called psychiatric physician trying to coerce others by pretending to be a healer combating a pestilential epidemic.

Some would cite the nastiness of the madman to justify the behavior of the psychiatrist. Others would cite the nastiness of the psychiatrist to justify the behavior of the madman. The upshot is that either madness or mad-doctoring is glamorized and romanticized, when, in fact, both are too often displays of deplorable behavior.

* * *

Communists seek to raise the poor above the rich, and justify their aim by claiming that the poor are noble, while the rich are corrupt. The motive of envy is concealed by the rhetoric of "liberation" from capitalist economic oppression.

* * *

Psychiatry

Anti-psychiatrists and radical psychiatrists (who are all self-declared socialists, communists, or at least anti-capitalists) seek to raise the "insane" above the "sane," and justify their aim by claiming that the "mentally ill" are authentic and honest, while the "mentally healthy" are inauthentic and corrupt. The motive of envy is now concealed by the rhetoric of "liberation" from capitalist psychiatric oppression.

* * *

Psychiatric diagnosis is a statement about the patient useful to the psychiatrist. Psychiatric symptom is a statement about the patient useful to the patient.

* * *

Under the guise of diagnosing disease, the psychiatrist disqualifies deviance.

* * *

The problem with psychiatric diagnoses is not that they are meaningless, but that they may be, and often are, swung as semantic blackjacks: cracking the subject's dignity and respectability destroys him just as effectively as cracking his skull. The difference is that the man who wields a blackjack is recognized by everyone as a thug, but one who wields a psychiatric diagnosis is not.

* * *

Psychiatric training is the ritualized indoctrination of the young physician into the theory and practice of psychiatric violence.

* * *

Traditional psychiatry distinguishes between minor and major mental illnesses (neuroses and psychoses), according to whether or not the patient has insight into his illness. Actually, psychiatrists classify a person as neurotic if he suffers from his problems in living, and as psychotic if he makes others suffer.

* * *

Psychiatrists say mental patients deny reality. I say that it is psychiatrists who deny reality, by calling unruly persons "mental patients" and their disturbing behavior "mental illness." For example: if a man goes to a bank and shoots the teller to steal money and so free himself from the oppression of poverty, that's called armed robbery; but if a man goes home and shoots his wife to kill her and so free himself from the oppression of marriage, that's called "temporary insanity."

* * *

Sadomasochistic sexual acts and involuntary psychiatric interventions have this in common: In the one, the male forces himself on a resisting female, gives her "pleasure" by appropriate sexual manipulation, and conceals his own domination and lust for orgasms behind his "partner's" dramatic orgastic response; in the other, the physician forces himself on a resisting "patient," gives him "treatment" by appropriate "medical" manipulations and conceals his own domination and lust for cures behind his "patient's" dramatic therapeutic response. In each case rape is justified by response.

* * *

Psychiatry

The organic psychiatrist believes that the brain "secretes delusions" just as the kidney secretes urine.

* * *

Community psychiatry promises to bring the day nearer when everyone will take care of everyone else, and no one will take care of himself.

* * *

In science, theories are constructed to fit facts; in forensic psychiatry, "facts" are constructed to fit theories. Or, put another way: in science theories are used to *explain* facts; in forensic psychiatry, they are used to *justify* actions.

* * *

The history of psychiatry, as recorded by psychiatrists and medical historians, proceeds from a faulty basic premise—namely, that the institutional psychiatrist helps and heals the involuntary patient. If Hitler had been victorious, the Germans could have written a similarly therapeutic account of the history of the concentration camps. Hence, there can be no popular appreciation of the true nature of the problem of mental illness until psychiatric histories are, so to speak, "denazified." "Great psychiatrists"—like Rush, Kraepelin, Alexander, Menninger, and even Pinel and Freud—must be seen as great leaders rather than as great healers. They helped their colleagues and the rulers of society, but harmed the madman and the victims of society.

Institutional Psychiatry

Institutional psychiatry comprises all psychiatric interventions and practices imposed on persons by others. These interventions are characterized by the complete loss of control by the client over his relationship with the expert—for example, in involuntary mental hospitalization. The most important economic characteristic of institutional psychiatry is that the institutional psychiatrist is a bureaucratic employee, paid for his services by a private or public organization (not by the individual who is his ostensible client). Its most important social characteristic is the use of force and fraud. The actual client of institutional psychiatry is some social interest and organization (for example, the Peace Corps, a university health service, a state mental hygiene department); its ostensible client is, more often than not, its victim rather than its beneficiary.

* * *

There are, and can be, no abuses *of* institutional psychiatry, because institutional psychiatry *is*, itself, an abuse, just as there were, and could be, no abuses *of* the

Inquisition, because the Inquisition *was,* itself, an abuse. Indeed, just as the Inquisition was the characteristic and perhaps inevitable abuse of Christianity, so institutional psychiatry is the characteristic and perhaps inevitable abuse of medicine.

* * *

The principal problem in institutional psychiatry is violence: the possible and feared violence of the madman, and the actual violence of society and the institutional psychiatrist against him.

* * *

The legitimacy of institutional psychiatry rests squarely on the dual premise that the "patients" lack self-control and are hence incapable of self-determination; and that the "therapists" not only possess these qualities, but are also professionally qualified experts in the "protection of the best interests of mentally sick patients."

* * *

Institutional psychiatry fulfills a basic human need—to validate the self as good (normal) by invalidating the other as evil (mentally ill).

* * *

The "depressive" is low on himself; the psychiatrist makes him high through drugs.

The "manic" is high on himself; the psychiatrist makes him low through drugs.

These examples illustrate the operating principle of institutional (and organic) psychiatry: Whatever the patient does is wrong, and whatever the psychiatrist does is right.

✲ ✲ ✲

Institutional psychiatry deals in judgments; psychoanalytic theory, in justifications.

Mental Hospitalization

Mental hospitals are the POW camps of our undeclared and inarticulated civil wars.

* * *

Voluntary mental hospitalization: the threat that "If you don't come quietly, it will only be harder on you" applied to persons accused of mental illness.

* * *

Involuntary mental hospitalization: according to mental hospital patients—indefinite imprisonment without crime, trial, or sentence; according to mental hospital psychiatrists—a practice so rare as to be practically nonexistent, resorted to solely for the protection of the mentally ill, and rejected only by those with paranoid fears of and hostilities toward institutional psychiatrists.

* * *

In fact, no person confined in a mental hospital is free to leave when he wants to. Nevertheless, the law distinguishes between two kinds of mental hospital patients: voluntary and involuntary. Voluntary patients *think* they can leave the hospital; involuntary patients *know* they cannot. The voluntary patient is wrong, and the involuntary patient right. Nevertheless, psychiatrists insist that voluntary patients suffer from mild mental diseases, and involuntary patients from serious ones, because the former have false beliefs convenient for the psychiatrist, while the latter have true beliefs inconvenient for him.

* * *

It has long been popular to bewail and denounce the inhumanity of incarcerating sane men in madhouses. To incarcerate so-called insane men is, in this view, permissible, because for them the "hospitalization" is a form of medical treatment, unpleasant to be sure, but always necessary and often helpful.

This view is wrong, and not only because there is no such thing as mental illness. It is wrong also because it is based on a fundamental misunderstanding of the medical ethic. In medicine a dangerous or mutilating intervention is permitted, not so much because it helps the sick person recover from his illness as because he wants it. For example, a patient with a cancerous lung may have a part of his lung removed. It would indeed be horrible if a surgeon did this to a person whose lung is perfectly healthy. But it would also be horrible if a surgeon did this to a cancerous patient against his will. For, in the final analysis, what makes a medical intervention morally permissible is not that it is therapeutic, but that it is something the patient wants. Similarly, what makes the quasi-medical intervention of involuntary psychiatric hospitalization morally impermissible is not that it is harmful, but that it is something the so-called patient does not want.

❋   ❋   ❋

Involuntary mental hospitalization is like slavery. Refining the standards for commitment is like prettifying the slave plantations. The problem is not how to improve commitment, but how to abolish it.

Psychoanalysis

Psychoanalysis is an attempt to examine a person's self-justifications. Hence it can be undertaken only with the patient's cooperation and can succeed only when the patient has something to gain by abandoning or modifying his system of self-justification.

* * *

The early Freudians believed that insight "cured." Later it was realized that it didn't, but psychoanalysts never explained what did. In the first place, it is senseless to speak of a cure where there is no disease. In the second place, insight stands in the same relationship to personality change as "is" stands to "ought," fact stands to value, or science stands to politics. This explains why insight cannot suffice to change anyone; and also why those who maintain that it is unnecessary in psychotherapy are as wrong as those who maintain that it is indispensable.

* * *

Whether psychoanalysis is or is not a science has been debated at length by philosophers, psychiatrists, and others. But the question is deceptive: the argument is, in fact, about whether psychoanalysis is good, true, or valid. Those who argue for the scientific basis of psychoanalysis affirm that it is "good," while those who argue against it deny this. This is an ironic confusion, first, because it rests on the tacit assumption that what is scientific is good; and second, because although psychoanalysis is not a science there is some good in it.

* * *

Freud said the hysteric "suffers from reminiscences." Not so. He suffers from his inability or refusal, in short his failure, to face and deal with his reminiscences. How else could the psychoanalyst help him?

* * *

Freud said religion was a neurosis. It would be more accurate to say that neurosis is a religion.

* * *

Freud never tired of asserting two contradictory claims: one, that it was not necessary that a person have medical or psychiatric qualifications to practice psychoanalysis; the other, that neuroses (and perversions, psychoses, etc.) were diseases. I think the reason for this was quite simple: on the one hand, he wanted to acquire the prestige and protection of medicine for the religious cult he was creating, and over which he wanted to rule—from the Berggasse while alive, and from the grave when dead; on the other hand, he knew, and realized that others would know, that conversation is not a form of medical treatment.

* * *

Free association: the term the psychoanalyst uses to register his approval of the patient who talks about what the analyst wants him to talk about. The opposite of resistance.

❖ ❖ ❖

Resistance: the term the psychoanalyst uses to register his disapproval of the patient who talks about what he himself wants to talk about rather than about what the analyst wants him to talk about.

❖ ❖ ❖

Libido theory: the litany of the Freudian services.

❖ ❖ ❖

Narcissist: psychoanalytic term for the person who loves himself more than his analyst; considered to be the manifestation of a dire mental disease whose successful treatment depends on the patient learning to love the analyst more and himself less.

❖ ❖ ❖

Psychoanalytic institute: a school where the faculty, composed of old and middle-aged men and women, called psychoanalysts, systematically degrade and infantilize the students, composed of psychiatrists themselves fast approaching middle age, who eagerly submit to this degradation ceremony in the expectation, often unfulfilled, that, after being completely deprived of all independent judgment and the capacity to form such judgment, they will be able to inflict a similar treatment on others, call it psychoanalysis, and charge high fees for it.

❖ ❖ ❖

The Second Sin

Psychoanalytic meetings: the Yom Kippur services of the secularized and "scientific" faithful: instead of regaling God in Hebrew with accounts of their own sinfulness, the worshipers regale each other, in the jargon of psychoanalysis, with accounts of the mental aberrations of their patients.

* * *

Psychoanalytic theory: the work song of the Freudian boatmen.

* * *

The unconscious: the "territory" of the psychoanalytic Mafia.

* * *

In psychoanalysis, the analyst's explanation of why other people act as they do is called "interpretation." Such explanations are basically of two types: those that analysts make about their patients to the patients themselves, and those they make about public figures to the general public.

The analyst's interpretations in the psychoanalytic situation conform to the general formula that the patient does not mean whatever he says or thinks he means—unless it is something bad. For example, when the patient says he loves his mother, father, or wife, that means he "really" hates them; but when he says he hates them, that also means he "really" hates them.

The analyst's interpretations outside of the psychoanalytic situation conform to the general formula that the subject is not what he appears to be or does not do what he appears to be doing—unless what he is or what he is doing is bad. For example, when the analyst interprets Leonardo da Vinci, he asserts that he was not "really" painting pictures but smearing feces; but when he interprets Oscar Wilde, he does not assert that Wilde was "really" a heterosexual.

* * *

When a man has sexual relations with many women, psychoanalysts say he has a Don Juan complex which signifies latent homosexuality. But when a man has sexual relations with many men, psychoanalysts do not say he has an Oscar Wilde complex which signifies latent heterosexuality. In short, the psychoanalytic vocabulary is rich in images and terms that demean and invalidate, and poor in those that dignify and validate.

* * *

In the jargon of psychoanalysis, rethinking and reexperiencing painful past experiences and memories with the goal of so ridding oneself of their lingering effects is called "working through." A major hazard of psychoanalysis (and of other forms of intensive psychotherapy) is that "working through" may become "reworking"; in other words, that instead of ridding himself of painful memories, the patient makes a career of ruminating about them and re-creating them in his present life. In short, aided and abetted by corrupt analysts, patients who have nothing better to do with their lives often use the psychoanalytic situation to transform insignificant childhood hurts into private shrines at which they worship unceasingly the enormity of the offenses committed against them. This solution is immensely flattering to the patients—as are all forms of unmerited self-aggrandizement; it is immensely profitable for the analysts—as are all forms pandering to people's vanity; and it is often immensely unpleasant for nearly everyone else in the patient's life.

* * *

The training analyst neither trains nor analyzes. He spies for the psychoanalytic institute that appoints him, and for the American Psychoanalytic Association, which accredits his institute. Thus does the model analyst become a symbol of all that is antithetical to the spirit of analysis. And thus does the training analysis, intended to purify and strengthen psychoanalysis, become the means of its pollution and destruction.

* * *

Beware of the psychoanalyst who analyzes jokes rather than laughs at them.

* * *

Psychoanalysis now functions as a religion disguised as a science and method of treatment. As Abraham received the Laws of God from Jehovah to whom he claimed to have had special access, so Freud received the Laws of Psychology from the Unconscious to which he claimed to have had special access.

* * *

"Words that are saturated with lies or atrocity," writes George Steiner, "do not easily resume life."[1] This is why the languages of madness and mad-doctoring are both dead languages. Each tries to deny its own mendacity:

[1] "K" (1963), in *Language and Silence: Essays on Language, Literature, and the Inhuman* (New York: Atheneum, 1967), p. 123.

the madman, through the fraudulent rhetoric of his "symptoms"; the mad doctor, through the fraudulent rhetoric of his "diagnoses" and "treatments."

Sartre, too, remarks on the role of the lie in the epistemology of psychoanalysis: "Thus psychoanalysis substitutes for the notion of bad faith the idea of a lie without a liar; it allows me to understand how it is possible for me to be lied to without lying to myself . . . ; it replaces the duality of the deceiver and the deceived, the essential condition of the lie, by that of the 'id' and the 'ego.' "[2]

But, in rehabilitating the lie, psychoanalysis annihilates the truth.

[2] Jean-Paul Sartre, *Being and Nothingness: An Essay on Phenomenological Ontology* (1943), translated by Hazel E. Barnes (New York: Philosophical Library, 1956), p. 51.

Mental Illness

Every "ordinary" illness that persons have, cadavers also have. A cadaver may thus be said to "have" cancer, pneumonia, or myocardial infarction. The only illness a cadaver surely cannot "have" is mental illness. Nevertheless, it is the official position of the American Medical Association, of the American Psychiatric Association, and of other medical and psychiatric groups that "mental illness is like any other illness."

* * *

Bodily illness is something the patient *has*, whereas mental illness is really something he *is* or *does*. If neurosis and psychosis were diseases, like pneumonia and cancer, it should be possible for a person to have *both* a neurosis and a psychosis. But the rules of psychiatric syntax make it absurd to assert such a diagnostic combination. Actually, we use the words "neurotic" and "psychotic" (and other psychiatric diagnostic terms) to characterize persons, not to name diseases.

* * *

Mental illness is a false definition of a problem abo
one's self and others. We don't say: "I live badly. I a
immoral"; instead we say: "I am confused. My min
doesn't work properly. I am sick." And we don't sa
"You live badly. You are immoral"; instead we say "Y(
are confused. Your mind doesn't work properly. You a
sick."

* * *

Mental illness is coercion concealed as loss of self-contr(
institutional psychiatry is countercoercion concealed .
therapy.

* * *

Mental illness is self-enhancing deception, self-promoti
strategy.

* * *

For the mental patient's family and society, mental illne
is a "problem"; for the patient himself it is a "solution
This was Freud's great discovery. Psychoanalysts no
ignore this, and psychiatrists deny it.

* * *

Much of what is called mental illness is habit—good (
bad, depending on who judges it and when. I sugge
this to a patient of mine who has had a long analysis wit
another therapist before coming to see me, and who h
"insight" into all that he is and is not doing. He sna
back: "I am not dropping a thirty-year pattern on a co
versation!"

* * *

Most of the things psychiatrists call "mental symptom
are actually declarations of independence and depen(

ence by the so-called mental patient. Characteristically, so-called psychotic symptoms are declarations of independence—that is, claims of increased powers and acquisition of control over self and others, as when a person asserts that he is Jesus; while so-called neurotic symptoms are declarations of dependence—that is, claims of decreased powers and loss of control over self and others, as when a person asserts that he is afraid of leaving the house or taking a job. It must be added that these declarations become symptoms, or are perceived as symptoms, only insofar as they are illegitimatized by the claimant's "loved ones" and by professionals in the mental health field.

* * *

Among persons categorized as mentally ill, there are two radically different types which are systematically undifferentiated by psychiatrists and hence confused by them. One is composed of the inadequate, unskilled, lazy, or stupid; in short, the unfit (however relative this term might be). The other of the protesters, the revolutionaries, those on strike against their relatives or society; in short, the unwilling.

Because they do not differentiate between these two groups, psychiatrists often attribute unfitness to unwillingness, and unwillingness to unfitness.

* * *

Parkinson's Law states that "Work expands so as to fill the time available for its completion."[1] Similarly, anxiety expands so as to fill the mental space available for its con-

[1] C. Northcote Parkinson, *Parkinson's Law, And Other Studies in Administration* (1957) (New York: Ballantine Books, 1964), p. 15.

templation. This is a restatement of the view that menta
disorders arise out of spiritual emptiness.

* * *

When a person's resistance against malevolent coercio
is at its lowest ebb; when he can no longer defend himsel
against intrusion by the other; he then suffers what i
popularly called a "nervous breakdown"; in psychiatri
jargon, he becomes "psychotic." He then claims eithe
that terrible things are happening to him (which is true)
or that he is invulnerably powerful (which is a sel
deception to make his life livable), or both.

* * *

We do not expect everyone to be a competent swimme
golfer, chess player, or marksman; nor do we regard thos
who play games poorly as "sick." The activities that con
prise being a student, parent, worker, etc. are, in man
ways, similar to the activities that comprise being a golf
or chess player. Yet we act as if we expected everyone t
play at his own life games competently; and we regar
those who play poorly—at being husband or wife, moth
or father—as "sick," that is, "mentally ill."

* * *

All belief and behavior is, among other things, an act
self-affirmation, as if the individual were asserting that
am the person that . . . believes that the Jews are th
Chosen People or that Jesus is the Son of God; is afra
of cancer or of crossing the street; etc." These sel
affirmations may please or annoy others, depending
their own values and relations to the individual maki

the claims, and on the measures the person has taken or promises to take to implement his beliefs. "Mental diseases" are members of a particular class of annoying self-affirmations.

* * *

If a man lies to us about his car so he can get more money from us, that is understandable economic behavior. But if he lies to us about himself so he can attract more attention to himself, that is mysterious madness. We respond to the former by bargaining about the price, and to the latter by fighting "mental illness."

* * *

The so-called mental patient makes statements and presents dramatizations which do not assert any facts, but rather command the onlooker to some sort of action. For example: The expansive, grandiose "schizophrenic" commands: "You must be subservient to me: I will help you, give you orders, etc." The agitated, self-accusatory "depressed" person commands: "You must dominate me: hate me, punish me, etc."

* * *

When a person does something bad, like shoot the President, it is immediately assumed that he might be mad—madness being thought of as a "disease" that might somehow "explain" why he did it. When a person does something good, like discover a cure for a hitherto incurable disease, no similar assumption is made. I submit that no further evidence is needed to show that "mental illness" is not the name of a biological condition whose nature awaits to be elucidated, but is the name of a concept whose purpose is to obscure the obvious.

* * *

Much of what passes for mental illness nowadays is actually the result of fearfulness and timidity. We speak of "the wages of sin," which are no doubt real enough. By the same token, we should speak of "the wages of fear": the fear to be, the fear to live and to die, the fear to be wrong, the fear to be envied or pitied, the fear to be different. Their wages are the multitudinous self-inhibitions we call mental illness.

* * *

Doubt is to certainty as neurosis is to psychosis. The neurotic is in doubt and has fears about persons and things; the psychotic has convictions and makes claims about them. In short, the neurotic has problems, the psychotic has solutions.

* * *

We say that a man "has" a neurosis or psychosis when we disagree with what he says or how he lives. We disguise this disagreement by attributing it to disease: if the patient were well, he would live as we do, not as he does. Voltaire was right: "If there were no God, it would be necessary to invent him." *Mutatis mutandis:* if there were no mental illness, it would be necessary to invent it.

* * *

In the nineteenth century psychiatrists were sometimes confronted by patients, usually women, who claimed they could not stand or walk, and when urged to try, would stagger in a dramatically clumsy way. They considered this a manifestation of the disease known as hysteria, and gave it the Greek-derived name "astasia-abasia." Actually, these patients were on strike against those who depended on their help; through body language, they said, in effect: "I can't get up and go out and do things with or for you." Had they simply said so, they would have felt guilty and would have also invited scorn and punishment, so they "converted" their message into hysterical symptoms.

The modern woman who becomes a housewife and feels herself a domestic slave displays the same sort of solution to the same conflict in her inability or fear to drive a car. Feeling duty-bound to do things for her family, she finds herself in the predicament of the competent slave: the more useful she becomes, the more she is, or feels herself, exploited. The less such a woman feels able to control the demands made upon her by her children and husband, the more she feels driven to claims of disability and incompetence as her sole protections against exploitation.

* * *

Conversion hysteria is to organic illness as counterfeit currency is to real money, or as a forged painting is to a genuine masterpiece.

* * *

Sartre says that hysteria is a lie without a liar. One could also say that the hysteric is a liar who does not admit or recognize his lies.

* * *

Phobia: a type of self-dramatization, as if the person were saying to himself: "I am afraid of X (cats, spiders, being alone, etc.), even though there is no reason to be afraid of X." His (or, more often, her) impoverished life thus becomes a kind of detective story, a cinematic thriller, or Grand Guignol. An empty life is thus transformed, without any real exertion or work, into a life full of interesting dangers, threats, and terrors. This solves the patient's problem of what to do with his life: he must protect himself from the dangers that threaten him.

* * *

Hypochondriasis: exaggerated attention to one's ill-health (real or pretended). The "illness" solves the problem of boredom and career choice: the hypochondriac is a Jeremiah of his own physiology.

* * *

The young adult who is afraid or refuses to build, we call "schizophrenic." The person who tries to live in someone else's house, we call "psychopathic" or "passive-dependent." The person who is contemptuous of what he has built, we call "depressed." The person who shows off his hovel as though it were a palace, we call "manic." Having diagnosed these mental diseases, we go off looking for the defective enzymes or twisted molecules in the so-called patient's brain. We claim we are looking for the causes of mental illness. Actually we are not trying to see anything, but on the contrary, are trying to blind ourselves to the tragedies of life that stare us in the eye. And in this we succeed remarkably well.

* * *

Mental illness as falsification:
Hysteria—the falsification of illness.
Schizophrenia—the falsification of meaning.
Psychopathy—the falsification of value.
Homosexuality, Transvestism—the falsification of gender role.

* * *

Mental illness as drama:
Depression—tragedy.
Mania—comedy.
Hysteria—melodrama.
Transvestism—farce.
Paranoia—parody.

* * *

Mental illness as caricature:
Depression—a caricature of contrition.
Hypochondriasis—a caricature of concern with one's health.
Mania—a caricature of love and devotion.
Paranoia—a caricature of concern with betrayal, danger, and protection.
Obsession and compulsion—a caricature of conscientiousness.

* * *

Today, particularly in the United States, all of the difficulties and problems of living are considered psychiatric diseases, and nearly everyone is considered to some extent mentally ill. Indeed, it is no exaggeration to say that life itself is now viewed as an illness that begins with conception and ends with death, requiring, at every step along the way, the skillful assistance of physicians and especially mental health professionals.

Myth of Mental Illness

Disease means bodily disease. Gould's Medical Diction-
ary defines disease as a disturbance of the function or
structure of an organ or a part of the *body*. The mind
(whatever it is) is not an organ or part of the body.
Hence, it cannot be diseased in the same sense as the
body can. When we speak of mental illness, then, we
speak metaphorically. To say that a person's mind is sick
is like saying that the economy is sick or that a joke is
sick. When metaphor is mistaken for reality and is used
for social purposes, then we have the makings of myth.
The concepts of mental health and mental illness are
mythological concepts, used strategically to advance
some social interests and to retard others, much as national and religious myths have been used in the past.

* * *

The myth of mental illness combines and confuses three
questions and the appropriate answers to each.

1. What *is it*: that is, what is the event, phenomenon,
or thing we are talking about? The answer is: it might be
brain disease, as in neurosyphilis; disapproved behavior,
as in depression; or the attribution of evil (called "bad-

ness" or "madness," "sin" or "sickness") to a scapegoa

2. What should we *call it:* that is, what name should w attach to the event, phenomenon, or thing we are obser ing and describing? The answer is: we might call it me tal illness or psychopathology; madness or genius; dev ance or disagreement; or psychiatric scapegoating.

3. How should we *treat it:* that is, what attitude policy should we adopt toward the event, phenomeno or thing—or the person regarded as its carrier? The a swer is: we might approve and reward it; disapprove an punish it; or remain neutral, tolerant, and essentially u responsive toward it.

In short, the contemporary mythology and rituals psychiatry make it virtually impossible for profession and layman alike to distinguish between phenomeno label, and policy. This explains, for example, the pe sistent belief that if the phenomena now often labele as schizophrenia were to be shown to be brain disease like neurosyphilis, that would justify the involuntary ps chiatric treatment of patients so diagnosed. But th would no more justify such treatment than would tl diagnosis of brain tumor justify the involuntary trea ment of persons afflicted with this disease.

* * *

Mental illness is a myth whose function is to disguise an thus render more palatable the bitter pill of moral co flicts in human relations. In asserting that there is no su thing as mental illness I do not deny that people hav problems coping with life and each other.

* * *

Bodily illness is to mental illness as literal meaning is to metaphorical meaning.

* * *

We may be dissatisfied with television for two quite different reasons: because our set does not work, or because we dislike the program we are receiving. Similarly, we may be dissatisfied with ourselves for two quite different reasons: because our body does not work (organic illness), or because we dislike our conduct (mental illness). How silly, wasteful, and destructive it would be if we would try to eliminate cigarette commercials from television by having TV repairmen work on our sets. How much more silly, wasteful, and destructive to try to eliminate phobias, and obsessions, and delusions, and what not by having psychiatrists work on our brains (with drugs, electroshock, and lobotomy).

* * *

Desires are aspirations we want to fulfill. Diseases are limitations we want to overcome. Two things could not be more unlike. Yet, in the hands of the modern psychiatrist, desires can become diseases. The desire for an abortion, a divorce, sexual embrace with a person of the same sex, prohibited drugs, and, of course, suicide—all of these are now widely considered to be mental diseases.

* * *

When I say that so-called mental illnesses are "problems in living," I mean only that they are matters of existence and meaning, not of health and disease. Freud knew this and said so when he acknowledged that his case histories read more like something that a novelist would write

111

than what a doctor would. That is exactly the point novelists write about how people live, and what the write is often largely autobiographical. When so-calle psychiatric patients tell their doctors the same sorts c "stories," the doctors conclude that people who live lik *that* must be sick and diagnose the patients as mentall ill. If this be diagnosis, it is the greatest folly of moder science.

Schizophrenia

If you talk to God, you are praying; if God talks to you, you have schizophrenia. If the dead talk to you, you are a spiritualist; if God talks to you, you are a schizophrenic.

* * *

When a man says that he is Jesus or Napoleon, or that the Martians are after him, or claims something else that seems outrageous to common sense, he is labeled psychotic and locked up in the madhouse.

Freedom of speech is only for normal people.

* * *

A man who says he is Jesus is not complaining, he is boasting. We consider his claim a symptom of illness; he considers it a stamp of greatness.

* * *

If you believe that you are Jesus, or have discovered a cure for cancer (and have not), or the Communists are after you (and they are not)—then your beliefs are likely to be regarded as symptoms of schizophrenia. But if you believe that the Jews are the Chosen People, or that Jesus was the Son of God, or that Communism is the only

scientifically and morally correct form of government—
then your beliefs are likely to be regarded as reflections
of who you are: Jew, Christian, Communist. This is
why I think that we will discover the chemical cause of
schizophrenia when we will discover the chemical cause
of Judaism, Christianity, and Communism. No sooner
and no later.

* * *

Psychiatrists look for twisted molecules and defective
genes as the causes of schizophrenia, because schizophrenia is the name of a disease. If Christianity or Communism were called diseases, would they then look for
the chemical and genetic "causes" of these "conditions"?

* * *

What we call schizophrenia is often the result of a certain
kind of the childhood development with respect to rule-
following. Normally, the child learns his basic repertory
of rules through loving submission to adult authority:
language, patterns of dress, and a great deal of everyday
conduct are learned in this way. If the adult is uncaring,
or is not respected by the child, we witness the development of the coercive megalomania so typical of the behavior of the person later diagnosed as schizophrenic.
This usually starts in the early teens. Not having a rule-
maker he can respect, the young person becomes his
own lawgiver. He acts and feels as if there were nothing
he could not do (especially if he tried hard enough)
and nothing he should not be allowed to do. And he
comes to believe that if he cannot do something, it must
not be worth doing. Such a person then tries to live not
by the rule that anything worth doing is worth doing

114

well, but by the maxim that only those things are worth
doing that he already knows how to do well; and since
he does not know how to do anything well, he alter-
nately pretends and claims mastery of arts, crafts, and
knowledge he does not possess; and scornfully rejects the
value of all practical endeavors. In short, (some) schizophrenia is a type of arrogance and immodesty.

* * *

Inflation is to money what schizophrenic word salad is to
language; each illustrates, first, that man is, in Nietzsche's
words, "an animal that makes promises," and second, that
it is easier to break promises than to keep them.

* * *

The "paranoid" hears, thinks, and claims that others are
mocking, ridiculing him, that is, that they are belittling
him, are diminishing his self-esteem. This is his justification for retaliating by mocking others and society. Ordinary man obeys the law of the land; the "paranoid" obeys
the commands of his own "higher law" (God, the voices
that talk to him) which order him to hate and to kill. In
his rejection of society's expectations, and in his inversion
of its rules, he revenges himself on his enemies.

* * *

The paranoid feels mocked, depreciated, because he is
mocked, depreciated—either by others or by his own valid
judgment of his failure in life.

Gerald Murphy (a friend of the Fitzgeralds) visits
Zelda in the Swiss sanatorium where she is confined by
Scott, and where she is reduced to basket weaving. He
describes his visit thus: "I moved as calmly as I could and

when I reached her I smiled and said that all my life had wanted to make baskets like hers—great, heavy stout baskets. . . . I stayed less than five minutes with her, but it was a harrowing experience."[1]

If men of letters treat madness with such profound self deception, what can one expect of people less given to reflecting on life?

* * *

Why have psychiatrists paid so much attention to the so called schizophrenic's symptoms, and so little to his rights Perhaps because many schizophrenics conduct them selves as if others had no rights: they violate thei privacy, not to mention their sense of reality. Hence, th schizophrenic may be treated as: 1. a dangerous mad man; 2. a person having highly dramatic and unusua experiences; or 3. a person disrespectful of the rights o others.

The first view is that of traditional psychiatry; the sec ond, that of the glamorizers of schizophrenia; the thir is my own.

* * *

When Jones says he is Jesus, scientific psychiatry declare him to have a delusion. I say he is lying. What is the dif ference? A delusion is something that happens to you that you "have." A lie is something you make happen something you do. Which view is correct? Something tha happens to a person—an accident or an error—is motiva tionally neutral: hence, it may be to the person's advan tage or disadvantage. But people with such delusion

[1] Nancy Milford, *Zelda: A Biography* (New York: Harper Row, 1970), p. 189.

never claim that they are Doe or Smith (their friends and neighbors); they always insist they are Jesus or Napoleon.

* * *

Some so-called paranoid delusions are, in effect, the expression of lack of courage. For example, the elderly woman who complains that her husband is poisoning her. She accuses. She complains. But she does not act. Why doesn't she kill him? Or leave him? Why doesn't she put her money where her mouth is? Because she lacks courage. She wants someone else to act on her belief, and be responsible for the consequences.

* * *

A woman in her fifties, whose husband died four years ago and whose children are grown and gone, has been put through electroshock, commitment, the works, by a large, extended family. She comes to see me of her own accord. What does she want? "They are poisoning me. They make funny remarks about me." And she smiles. When I suggest that she might prefer to think that to thinking that her life is empty and meaningless, she says: "If you would only know how they hurt me. . . ." A fleeting smile remains on her face. The so-called inappropriate affect—what psychiatrists consider the classic symptom of schizophrenia—is perhaps the poorly suppressed amusement of the con man, secretly laughing at his mark.

Psychology

There is no psychology; there is only biography and autobiography.

* * *

Before the bar of justice, ignorance of the law is no excuse. Before the bar of psychology, ignorance of history is not only an excuse but a requirement for recognition.

* * *

Intelligence tests: hocus-pocus used by psychologists to prove that they are brilliant, and their clients stupid. The general acceptance of these tests suggests that this claim may not be without foundation.

* * *

Projective tests: hocus-pocus used by psychologists to prove that they are normal and that their clients are crazy. The popular acceptance of these tests suggests that this claim, too, may not be without foundation.

* * *

Personality theory: familial and social policies disguised as empirical observations and promoted as scientific laws.

* * *

Freudian psychology is the psychology of the adolescent male: sex-starved and sex-crazed, seeing the world in terms of sexual frustrations and satisfactions.

Adlerian psychology is the psychology of the young adult male: craving control and power, seeing the world in terms of dominance and submission.

Jungian psychology is the psychology of the middle-aged person, man and woman: longing for religion but unable to believe, seeing the world in terms of infinite varieties of meanings and mysteries.

Psychotherapy

Psychotherapy is the name we give to a particular kind of personal influence: by means of communications, one person, identified as "the psychotherapist," exerts an ostensibly therapeutic influence on another, identified as "the patient." It is evident, however, that this process is but a special member of a much larger class—indeed, of a class so vast that virtually all human interactions fall within it. Not only in psychotherapy, but also in countless other situations, such as advertising, education, friendship, and marriage, people influence one another. Who is to say whether such interactions are helpful or harmful, and to whom? The concept of psychotherapy betrays us on this point by prejudging the interaction as therapeutic for the patient, in intent or effect or both.

* * *

People seeking help from psychotherapists can be divided into two groups: those who wish to confront their difficulties and shortcomings and change their lives by changing themselves; and those who wish to avoid the inevitable consequences of their life strategies through the magical or tactical intervention of the therapist in their lives. Those in the former group may derive great benefit from therapy in a few weeks or months; those in the latter may stand still, or sink ever deeper into their self-created life morass, after meeting with psycho-therapists for years, and even decades.

* * *

In most types of voluntary psychothherapy, the therapist tries to elucidate the inexplicit game rules by which the client conducts himself; and to help the client scrutinize the goals and values of the life games he plays.

* * *

Success in psychotherapy—that is, the ability to change oneself in a direction in which one wants to change—re-quires courage rather than insight.

* * *

Autonomous psychotherapy is characterized by its aim—to increase the client's knowledge of himself and others and hence his freedom of choice in the conduct of his life; by its method—the analysis of communications, rules and games; and by its social context—a contractual, rather than a therapeutic, relationship between analyst and analysand.

* * *

The autonomous psychotherapist's role vis-à-vis his client is like the court jester's vis-à-vis the monarch: therapist confronts client with painful reality, but in as friendly a way as possible; client retains all the power over whether he wants to listen or not (that is, whether he wants to continue or terminate the therapeutic relationship).

* * *

People with personal problems often behave like the proverbial drunk who looks for his house key under the streetlight, not because that's where he dropped it, but because that's where the light is. Should such a person consult an autonomous psychotherapist, the therapist's job is not to try to find the key, but to suggest to the "patient" that he light a match or borrow a flashlight from a neighbor and go look for his key where he dropped it.

* * *

"Hard cases make bad law" is a sound legal maxim. *Mutatis mutandis:* desperate clients make bad psychotherapy. Sound and sensible rules for psychotherapy must rest on a contract between a client able to inspect his own life and learn from his mistakes, and a psychotherapist competent to help him with this task. Desperately distraught clients often suffer from the consequences of their stupidity compounded by their stubbornness; and they often succeed in provoking a matching set of stupid and stubborn responses in their psychiatrists—which the latter rationalize and even glorify as "emergency methods of psychotherapy."

* * *

When people (especially women) consult psychotherapists, they are often on the brink of having to choose between two conflicting life strategies; that is, between increasing their self-pity, by appearing helpless and victimized, to extort from others what they feel they need; and increasing their self-esteem, by becoming more competent and self-reliant, to provide for themselves what they decide they want.

* * *

Psychotherapies (and all so-called psychiatric treatments) should be viewed as analogous to sexual relations, and should be so regulated by the state: So long as they are consensual—that is, so long as both (or all) parties engaging in the "therapy" are satisfied with it—it should be permissible; and it should be no one else's business whether it's good or bad ("therapeutic" or "noxious"). Involuntary psychiatric therapy, like rape, should be prohibited and punished by the criminal law.

* * *

Hypnosis: two people lying to each other, each pretending to believe both his own and his partner's lies.

Professionalism

Paternalism: the moral principle that enjoins a person to give another everything but respect. The doctrine according to which no one is yet ready for freedom and self-determination except the speaker and the group of which he is a member. The foundation of professionalism.

*   *   *

Someone once defined a psychoanalyst as a nonswimmer working as a lifeguard. True enough, often enough. Most professionals are nonswimmers working as lifeguards. Professionalization is certifying nonswimmers as lifeguards, and preventing swimmers from working as lifeguards.

*   *   *

The double standard in sex, discriminating between men and women—on the ancient principle of *Quod licet Jovi, non licet bovi* (What is permitted to Jove, is not permitted to the cow)—has an analogue in the even more hypocritical and pervasive double standard between the expert and the layman. The sexual double standard says that men are virile and women are nymphomaniacs. The professional double standard says that the experts are sexologists and therapists, while the laymen are pornographers, pimps, and prostitutes; the experts are physicians and methadone-maintenance researchers, the laymen are pushers and corrupters of the nation; the experts are skeptical and demand proof, the laymen are suspicious and suffer from paranoia.

❆ ❆ ❆

Birth and death, the two most natural and "normal" biological occurrences, have become preempted by the medical profession. Thus pregnancy and senility are regarded as diseases whose management requires expert medical assistance. It is small wonder that the medical profession tyrannizes over the everyday life of a people who refuse to take responsibility for the most elementary tasks their biological makeup poses for them.

❆ ❆ ❆

Being judged by a professional colleague is like betting with a person who follows the rule: "Heads I win, tails you lose." If your facts or reasoning are wrong, he will prove you wrong by marshaling the true facts and correct reasoning; and if your facts and reasoning are right, he will prove you wrong by attributing immoralities to your character and mental diseases to your personality.

Science and Scientism

he essence of the scientific enterprise is the effort to
nderstand something in order better to control it. In
atural science, this means that the scientist, man, stud-
s and controls the object of his interest, a thing. The
ing studied has no say in this matter. Hence, the moral
mensions and dilemmas of natural science derive not
om a conflict between the scientist and the object he
udies, but from a conflict between the scientist and
her persons or groups who may disapprove of the per-
nal and social consequences of his work.

In human or moral science (if it may be called a
cience") the situation is radically different. Here, the
ientist, man, studies and controls the object of his in-
rest, a person. The subject studied is very much con-
rned with this process. Hence, the moral dimensions
d dilemmas of human science derive from two distinct
urces: first, from a conflict between scientist and sub-
ct, and second, from a conflict between scientist and
her persons or groups who may disapprove of the per-
nal and social consequences of his work.

In short, although both the natural and moral sciences

seek to understand the objects of their observation,
natural science the purpose of this is to be able to cont
them better, whereas in moral science it is, or ought
be, to be better able to leave them alone. The mora
proper aim of psychology, then, is self-control.

* * *

Formerly, when religion was strong and science we
men mistook magic for medicine; now, when science
strong and religion weak, men mistake medicine
magic.

* * *

Psychiatry is institutionalized scientism: it is system
imitation, impersonation, counterfeiting, and decepti
This is the formula: every adult smokes (drinks,
gages in sexual activity, etc.); hence, to prove that he
an adult, the adolescent smokes (drinks, engages in s
ual activity, etc.). *Mutatis mutandis:* every science c
sists of classification, control, and prediction; hence,
prove that psychiatry is a science, the psychiatrist cl
sifies, controls, and predicts. The result is that he classi
people as mad; that he confines people as dangerous
themselves or others); and that he predicts people's
havior, robbing them of their free will and hence of th
very humanity.

* * *

For the Jews, the Messiah has never come; for the Ch
tians, He has come but once; for modern man, He
pears and disappears with increasing rapidity. T
saviors of modern man, the "scientists" who promise s

vation through the "discoveries" of ethology and sociology, psychology and psychiatry, and all the other bogus religions, issue forth periodically, as if selected by some Messiah-of-the-Month Club.

Therapeutic State

A Theological State is characterized, among other things, by the preoccupation of its people with religion in general, and with heresy in particular. Similarly, a Therapeutic State is characterized, among other things, by the preoccupation of its people with health in general, and with quackery in particular. *Mutatis mutandis,* as in a society with religious freedom the concept of heresy loses its significance, so in a society with medical freedom the concept of quackery would lose its significance. The very absurdity of the latter prospect is a measure of the depth of our reliance on the state for the protection of our bodies—a reliance wholly analogous to that of our ancestors on the church for the protection of their souls.

* * *

Freedom of religion means freedom from religious domination and persecution. Similarly, freedom of medicine means freedom from medical domination and persecution. As the one has required a separation of church and state, so the other requires a separation of medicine and the state.

If we truly value medical healing and refuse to confuse

it with therapeutic oppression—as the Founding Fathe
truly valued religious faith and refused to confuse it wi
theological oppression—then we ought to let each ma
seek his own medical salvation and erect an invisible b
impenetrable wall separating medicine and the state.

* * *

We have no national religion. Neither do the Russian
But both the U.S.A. and the U.S.S.R. (and many oth
modern nations) have national, or state-recognized an
state-supported, medicine. This corrupts medicine in tl
same way as religion had formerly been corrupted by i
alliance with the state. Although the existence of th
corruption is widely recognized, its cause is usually a
tributed to too little, rather than too much, control b
the state. To return medicine to the service of the i
dividual nothing less will suffice than an extension of tl
protections of the First Amendment to the healing art
guaranteeing that "Congress shall make no law respec
ing an establishment of medicine, or prohibiting the fre
exercise thereof. . . ."

* * *

The First Amendment protects religious freedom, yet th
Mormons are forbidden to practice polygamy. Since pr
gressive opinion now holds that medical treatment is
right, the Mormons ought to claim that they need sever
wives for their mental health rather than for their rel
gious well-being. Then, like heroin addicts who are sai
to have a "right" to methadone, Mormons might obtai
the "right" to polygamy.

* * *

Christian Science denies illness; it defines and perceives sickness as sin.

Atheist Science denies evil; it defines and perceives sin as sickness.

Actually, both sickness and sin, illness and evil, exist and are real. We often confuse them in order to confuse, and thereby to control, others.

* * *

Medignosis: the doctrine that all human problems are medical diseases curable by appropriate therapeutic interventions, imposed on the patient by force if necessary. The "scientific" successor of pre-Christian and Christian forms of gnosticism; the dominant religious faith of modern man.

* * *

Bad habits treated as diseases:

Using alcohol badly is called "alcoholism" and is treated with Antabuse.

Using food badly is called "anorexia nervosa" or "obesity"; the former is treated with electroshock, the latter with amphetamines or intestinal bypass operation.

Using sex badly is called perversion, and is treated with stimulation through electrodes implanted in the brain and with sex-change operations.

Using language badly is called "schizophrenia" and is treated with lobotomy.

* * *

Therapeutism: the successor to patriotism. The last refuge—or the first, depending on the authority consulted —of scoundrels. The creed that justifies proclaiming un-

133

dying love for those we hate, and inflicting merciless punishment on them in the name of treating them for diseases whose principal symptoms are their refusal to submit to our domination.

* * *

We live in an age characterized by a tremendous need for vast numbers of mental patients upon whom, as products or things, a large part of the rest of the population can work, and which those considered mentally healthy can proudly support. The result is the Therapeutic State, whose aim is not to provide favorable conditions for life, liberty, and the pursuit of happiness, but to repair the defective mental health of its citizens. The officials of such a state parody the roles of physician and psychotherapist. This arrangement gives meaning to the lives of countless bureaucrats, physicians, and mental health workers by robbing the so-called patients of the meaning of their lives. We thus persecute millions—as drug addicts, homosexuals, suicidal risks, and so forth—all the while telling ourselves that we are great healers, curing them of mental illness. We have managed to repackage the Inquisition and are selling it as a new, scientific cure all.

* * *

Man's domination over his fellow man is as old as history and we may safely assume that it is traceable to prehistoric times and to prehuman ancestors. Perennially, men have oppressed women; white men, colored men; Christians, Jews. However, in recent decades, traditional reasons and justifications for discrimination among men—on the grounds of national, racial, or religious criteria—

have lost much of their plausibility and appeal. What justification is there now for man's age-old desire to dominate and control his fellow man? Modern liberalism—in reality, a type of statism—allied with scientism, has met the need for a fresh defense of oppression and has supplied a new battle cry: health!

In this therapeutic-meliorist view of society, the ill form a special class of "victims" who must, both for their own good and for the interests of the community, be "helped"—coercively and against their will, if necessary—by the healthy, and especially by physicians who are "scientifically" qualified to be their masters. This perspective developed first and has advanced furthest in psychiatry, where the oppression of "insane patients" by "sane physicians" is by now a social custom hallowed by medical and legal tradition. At present, the medical profession as a whole seems to be emulating this model. In the Therapeutic State toward which we appear to be moving, the principal requirement for the position of Big Brother may be an M.D. degree.